ABC OF HEART FAILURE

ABC OF HEART FAILURE

Edited by

CHRISTOPHER R GIBBS
Research Fellow
University Department of Medicine and Department of Cardiology
City University, Birmingham

MICHAEL K DAVIES
Consultant Cardiologist
Department of Cardiology, Selly Oak Hospital, Birmingham

and

GREGORY Y H LIP
Consultant Cardiologist and Reader in Medicine
University Department of Medicine and Department of Cardiology
City Hospital, Birmingham

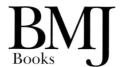
BMJ
Books

© BMJ Books 2000
BMJ Books is an imprint of the BMJ Publishing Group

First published in 2000
Second impression in 2001
Third impression in 2001
Fourth impression in 2002
by BMJ Books, BMA House, Tavistock Square,
London WC1H 9JR

www.bmjbooks.com

British Library Cataloguing in Publication Data
A catalogue record for this book is available from the British Library

ISBN 0-7279-1457-X

Composition by Scribe Design, Gillingham, Kent
Printed and bound in Spain by GraphyCems, Navarra

Contents

Contributors

DG Beevers
Professor of Medicine, University Department of Medicine and Department of Cardiology, City Hospital, Birmingham

MK Davies
Consultant Cardiologist, Department of Cardiology, Selly Oak Hospital, Birmingham

RC Davis
Clinical Research Fellow, Department of Primary Care and General Practice, University of Birmingham

CR Gibbs
Research Fellow, University Department of Medicine and Department of Cardiology, City University, Birmingham

FDR Hobbs
Professor, Department of Primary Care and General Practice, University of Birmingham

G Jackson
Consultant Cardiologist, Department of Cardiology, Guy's and St Thomas' Hospital, London

GYH Lip
Consultant Cardiologist and Reader in Medicine, University Department of Medicine and Department of Cardiology, City Hospital, Birmingham

T Millane
Consultant Cardiologist, Department of Cardiology, City Hospital, Birmingham

RDS Watson
Consultant Cardiologist, University Department of Medicine and Department of Cardiology, City Hospital, Birmingham

Preface

The epidemiology, diagnosis and management of heart failure have changed significantly over the last decade. Heart failure is now a major cause of morbidity and mortality, estimated to account for many admissions to hospital and attendances in general practices. The overall incidence is likely to increase even further in the future, with an ageing population and, paradoxically, with therapeutic advances in the management of myocardial infarction leading to improved survival but potentially leaving many patients with impaired cardiac function which may subsequently progress. Unfortunately. heart failure can be very difficult to diagnose clinically, since many features are not specific to the disease, and there may be few symptoms or clinical signs especially in the early stages of the disease.

However, recent therapeutic advances have made the early recognition of heart failure increasingly important. The ACE inhibitors are now central to therapy for heart failure, both in symptomatic cases and asymptomatic left ventricular dysfunction. Many of today's clinicians will remember being taught as medical students that beta-blockers are absolutely contraindicated in heart failure, but recent trials have clearly demonstrated a significant benefit of these agents in chronic heart failure. Furthermore, the use of the aldosterone antagonist, spironolactone. in combination with ACE inhibitors was considered potentially dangerous, until a recent trial showing the additive effects of both these agents in inhibiting neuroendocrine activation in heart failure, with few side effects.

The *ABC of Heart Failure* intends to be a clear practical guide and to provide a basis for a greater understanding of the disease, its investigation and practical management. The main challenge is to ensure that validated treatments are given to all who need it. We hope that the series published in the BMJ and this book would heighten awareness of this devastating condition, which if untreated can have a prognosis worse than many forms of cancer, and help improve its management in both hospital and general practice.

Christopher R Gibbs
Michael K Davis
Gregory YH Lip

1 History and epidemiology

R C Davis, F D R Hobbs, G Y H Lip

Heart failure is the end stage of all diseases of the heart and is a major cause of morbidity and mortality. It is estimated to account for about 5% of admissions to hospital medical wards, with over 100 000 annual admissions in the United Kingdom.

The overall prevalence of heart failure is 3-20 per 1000 population, although this exceeds 100 per 1000 in those aged 65 years and over. The annual incidence of heart failure is 1-5 per 1000, and the relative incidence doubles for each decade of life after the age of 45 years. The overall incidence is likely to increase in the future, because of both an ageing population and therapeutic advances in the management of acute myocardial infarction leading to improved survival in patients with impaired cardiac function.

Unfortunately, heart failure can be difficult to diagnose clinically, as many features of the condition are not organ specific, and there may be few clinical features in the early stages of the disease. Recent advances have made the early recognition of heart failure increasingly important as modern drug treatment has the potential to improve symptoms and quality of life, reduce hospital admission rates, slow the rate of disease progression, and improve survival. In addition, coronary revascularisation and heart valve surgery are now regularly performed, even in elderly patients.

A brief history

Descriptions of heart failure exist from ancient Egypt, Greece, and India, and the Romans were known to use the foxglove as medicine. Little understanding of the nature of the condition can have existed until William Harvey described the circulation in 1628. Röntgen's discovery of *x* rays and Einthoven's development of electrocardiography in the 1890s led to improvements in the investigation of heart failure. The advent of echocardiography, cardiac catheterisation, and nuclear medicine have since improved the diagnosis and investigation of patients with heart failure.

Blood letting and leeches were used for centuries, and William Withering published his account of the benefits of digitalis in 1785. In the 19th and early 20th centuries, heart failure associated with fluid retention was treated with Southey's tubes, which were inserted into oedematous peripheries, allowing some drainage of fluid.

> **"The very essence of cardiovascular practice is the early detection of heart failure"**
> **Sir Thomas Lewis, 1933**

Some definitions of heart failure

"A condition in which the heart fails to discharge its contents adequately" (Thomas Lewis, 1933)

"A state in which the heart fails to maintain an adequate circulation for the needs of the body despite a satisfactory filling pressure" (Paul Wood, 1950)

"A pathophysiological state in which an abnormality of cardiac function is responsible for the failure of the heart to pump blood at a rate commensurate with the requirements of the metabolising tissues" (E Braunwald, 1980)

"Heart failure is the state of any heart disease in which, despite adequate ventricular filling, the heart's output is decreased or in which the heart is unable to pump blood at a rate adequate for satisfying the requirements of the tissues with function parameters remaining within normal limits" (H Denolin, H Kuhn, H P Krayenbuehl, F Loogen, A Reale, 1983)

"A clinical syndrome caused by an abnormality of the heart and recognised by a characteristic pattern of haemodynamic, renal, neural and hormonal responses" (Philip Poole-Wilson, 1985)

"[A] syndrome ... which arises when the heart is chronically unable to maintain an appropriate blood pressure without support" (Peter Harris, 1987)

"A syndrome in which cardiac dysfunction is associated with reduced exercise tolerance, a high incidence of ventricular arrhythmias and shortened life expectancy" (Jay Cohn, 1988)

"Abnormal function of the heart causing a limitation of exercise capacity" or "ventricular dysfunction with symptoms" (anonymous and pragmatic)

"Symptoms of heart failure, objective evidence of cardiac dysfunction and response to treatment directed towards heart failure" (Task Force of the European Society of Cardiology, 1995)

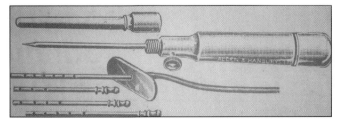

Southey's tubes were at one time used for removing fluid from oedematous peripheries in patients with heart failure

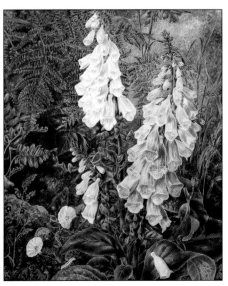

The foxglove was used as a medicine in heart disease as long ago as Roman times

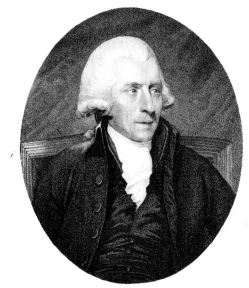

In 1785 William Withering of Birmingham published an account of medicinal use of digitalis

A brief history of heart failure

1628	William Harvey describes the circulation
1785	William Withering publishes an account of medical use of digitalis
1819	René Laennec invents the stethoscope
1895	Wilhelm Röntgen discovers x rays
1920	Organomercurial diuretics are first used
1954	Inge Edler and Hellmuth Hertz use ultrasound to image cardiac structures
1958	Thiazide diuretics are introduced
1967	Christiaan Barnard performs first human heart transplant
1987	CONSENSUS-I study shows unequivocal survival benefit of angiotensin converting enzyme inhibitors in severe heart failure
1995	European Society of Cardiology publishes guidelines for diagnosing heart failure

It was not until the 20th century that diuretics were developed. The early, mercurial agents, however, were associated with substantial toxicity, unlike the thiazide diuretics, which were introduced in the 1950s. Vasodilators were not widely used until the development of angiotensin converting enzyme inhibitors in the 1970s. The landmark CONSENSUS-I study (first cooperative north Scandinavian enalapril survival study), published in 1987, showed the unequivocal survival benefits of enalapril in patients with severe heart failure.

Epidemiology

Studies of the epidemiology of heart failure have been complicated by the lack of universal agreement on a definition of heart failure, which is primarily a clinical diagnosis. National and international comparisons have therefore been difficult, and mortality data, postmortem studies, and hospital admission rates are not easily translated into incidence and prevalence. Several different systems have been used in large population studies, with the use of scores for clinical features determined from history and examination, and in most cases chest radiography, to define heart failure.

The Task Force on Heart Failure of the European Society of Cardiology has recently published guidelines on the diagnosis of heart failure, which require the presence of symptoms and objective evidence of cardiac dysfunction. Reversibility of symptoms on appropriate treatment is also desirable. Echocardiography is recommended as the most practicable way of assessing cardiac function, and this investigation has been used in more recent studies.

In the Framingham heart study a cohort of 5209 subjects has been assessed biennially since 1948, with a further cohort (their offspring) added in 1971. This uniquely large dataset has been used to determine the incidence and prevalence of heart failure, defined with consistent clinical and radiographic criteria.

Several recent British studies of the epidemiology of heart failure and left ventricular dysfunction have been conducted, including a study of the incidence of heart failure in one west London district (Hillingdon heart failure study) and large prevalence studies in Glasgow (north Glasgow MONICA study) and the West Midlands ECHOES (echocardiographic heart of England screening) study. It is important to note that

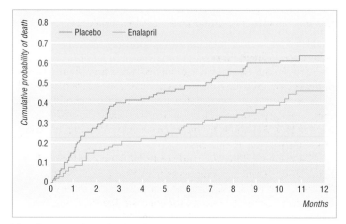

Mortality curves from the CONSENSUS-I study

The Framingham heart study has been the most important longitudinal source of data on the epidemiology of heart failure

Contemporary studies of the epidemiology of heart failure in United Kingdom

Study	Diagnostic criteria
Hillingdon heart failure study (west London)	Clinical (for example, shortness of breath, effort intolerance, fluid retention), radiographic, and echocardiographic
ECHOES study (West Midlands)	Clinical and echocardiographic (ejection fraction <40%)
MONICA population (north Glasgow)	Clinical and echocardiographic (ejection fraction ≤30%)

epidemiological studies of heart failure have used different levels of ejection fraction to define systolic dysfunction. The Glasgow study, for example, used an ejection fraction of 30% as their criteria, whereas most other epidemiological surveys have used levels of 40-45%. Indeed, prevalence of heart failure seems similar in many different surveys, despite variation in the levels of ejection fraction, and this observation is not entirely explained.

Prevalence of heart failure

During the 1980s the Framingham study reported the age adjusted overall prevalence of heart failure, with similar rates for men and women. Prevalence increased dramatically with increasing age, with an approximate doubling in the prevalence of heart failure with each decade of ageing.

In Nottinghamshire, the prevalence of heart failure in 1994 was estimated from prescription data for loop diuretics and examination of the general practice notes of a sample of these patients, to determine the number who fulfilled predetermined criteria for heart failure. The overall prevalence of heart failure was estimated as 1.0% to 1.6%, rising from 0.1% in the 30-39 age range to 4.2% at 70-79 years. This method, however, may exclude individuals with mild heart failure and include patients treated with diuretics who do not have heart failure.

Incidence of heart failure

The Framingham data show an age adjusted annual incidence of heart failure of 0.14% in women and 0.23% in men. Survival in the women is generally better than in the men, leading to the same point prevalence. There is an approximate doubling in the incidence of heart failure with each decade of ageing, reaching 3% in those aged 85-94 years.

The recent Hillingdon study examined the incidence of heart failure, defined on the basis of clinical and radiographic findings, with echocardiography, in a population in west London. The overall annual incidence was 0.08%, rising from 0.02% at age 45-55 years to 1.2% at age 86 years or over. About 80% of these cases were first diagnosed after acute hospital admission, with only 20% being identified in general practice and referred to a dedicated clinic.

The Glasgow group of the MONICA study and the ECHOES Group have found that coronary artery disease is the most powerful risk factor for impaired left ventricular function, either alone or in combination with hypertension. In these studies hypertension alone did not appear to contribute substantially to impairment of left ventricular systolic contraction, although the Framingham study did report a more substantial contribution from hypertension. This apparent difference between the studies may reflect improvements in the treatment of hypertension and the fact that some patients with hypertension, but without coronary artery disease, may develop heart failure as a result of diastolic dysfunction.

Prevalence of left ventricular dysfunction

Large surveys have been carried out in Britain in the 1990s, in Glasgow and the West Midlands, using echocardiography.

In Glasgow the prevalence of significantly impaired left ventricular contraction in subjects aged 25-74 years was 2.9%; in the West Midlands, the prevalence was 1.8% in subjects aged 45 and older.

The higher rates in the Scottish study may reflect the high prevalence of ischaemic heart disease, the main precursor of impaired left ventricular function in both studies. The numbers of symptomatic and asymptomatic cases, in both studies, were about the same.

Prevalence of heart failure (per 1000 population), Framingham heart study

Age (years)	Men	Women
50-59	8	8
80-89	66	79
All ages	7.4	7.7

Methods of assessing prevalence of heart failure in published studies

- Clinical and radiographic assessment
- Echocardiography
- General practice monitoring
- Drug prescription data

Annual incidence of heart failure (per 1000 population), Framingham heart study

Age (years)	Men	Women
50-59	3	2
80-89	27	22
All ages	2.3	1.4

The MONICA study is an international study conducted under the auspices of the World Health Organisation to monitor trends in and determinants of mortality from cardiovascular disease

---

Prevalence (%) of left ventricular dysfunction, north Glasgow (MONICA survey)

Age group (years)	Asymptomatic		Symptomatic	
	Men	Women	Men	Women
45-54	4.4	1.2	1.4	1.2
55-64	3.2	0.0	2.5	2.0
65-74	3.2	1.3	3.2	3.6

Ethnic differences

Ethnic differences in the incidence of and mortality from heart failure have also been reported. In the United States, African-American men have been reported as having a 33% greater risk of being admitted to hospital for heart failure than white men; the risk for black women was 50%.

A similar picture emerged in a survey of heart failure among acute medical admissions to a city centre teaching hospital in Birmingham. The commonest underlying aetiological factors were coronary heart disease in white patients, hypertension in black Afro-Caribbean patients, and coronary heart disease and diabetes in Indo-Asians. Some of these racial differences may be related to the higher prevalence of hypertension and diabetes in black people and coronary artery disease and diabetes mellitus in Indo-Asians.

Impact on health services

Heart failure accounts for at least 5% of admissions to general medical and geriatric wards in British hospitals, and admission rates for heart failure in various European countries (Sweden, Netherlands, and Scotland) and in the United States have doubled in the past 10-15 years. Furthermore, heart failure accounts for over 1% of the total healthcare expenditure in the United Kingdom, and most of these costs are related to hospital admissions. The cost of heart failure is increasing, with an estimated UK expenditure in 1996 of £465m (£556m when the costs of community health services and nursing homes are included).

Hospital readmissions and general practice consultations often occur soon after the diagnosis of heart failure. In elderly patients with heart failure, readmission rates range from 29-47% within 3 to 6 months of the initial hospital discharge. Treating patients with heart failure with angiotensin converting enzyme inhibitors can reduce the overall cost of treatment (because of reduced hospital admissions) despite increased drug expenditure and improved long term survival.

The pictures of William Withering and of the foxglove are reproduced with permission from the Fine Art Photographic Library. The box of definitions of heart failure is adapted from Poole-Wilson PA et al, eds (*Heart failure.* New York: Churchill Livingstone, 1997:270). The table showing the prevalence of left ventricular dysfunction in north Glasgow is reproduced with permission from McDonagh TA et al (see key references box). The table showing costs of heart failure is adapted from McMurray J et al (*Br J Med Econ* 1993;6:99-110).

In the United States mortality from heart failure at age <65 years has been reported as being up to 2.5-fold higher in black patients than in white patients

Cost of heart failure

Country	Cost	% Healthcare costs	% Of costs due to admissions
UK, 1990-1	£360m	1.2	60
US, 1989	$9bn	1.5	71
France, 1990	FF11.4bn	1.9	64
New Zealand, 1990	$NZ73m	1.5	68
Sweden, 1996	Kr2.6m	2.0	75

Key references

- Clarke KW, Gray D, Hampton JR. Evidence of inadequate investigation and treatment of patients with heart failure. *Br Heart J* 1994;71:584-7.
- Cowie MR, Mosterd A, Wood DA, Deckers JW, Poole-Wilson PA, Sutton GC, et al. The epidemiology of heart failure. *Eur Heart J* 1997;18:208-25.
- Cowie MR, Wood DA, Coats AJS, Thompson SG, Poole-Wilson PA, Suresh V, et al. Incidence and aetiology of heart failure: a population-based study. *Eur Heart J* 1999;20:421-8.
- Dries DL, Exner DV, Gersh BJ, Cooper HA, Carson PE, Domanski MJ. Racial differences in the outcome of left ventricular dysfunction. *N Engl J Med* 1999;340:609-16.
- Ho KK, Pinsky JL, Kannel WB, Levy D. The epidemiology of heart failure: the Framingham study. *J Am Coll Cardiol* 1993;22:6-13A.
- Lip GYH, Zarifis J, Beevers DG. Acute admissions with heart failure to a district general hospital serving a multiracial population. *Int J Clin Pract* 1997;51:223-7.
- McDonagh TA, Morrison CE, Lawrence A, Ford I, Tunstall-Pedoe H, McMurray JJV, et al. Symptomatic and asymptomatic left-ventricular systolic dysfunction in an urban population. *Lancet* 1997;350:829-33.
- The Task Force on Heart Failure of the European Society of Cardiology. Guidelines for the diagnosis of heart failure. *Eur Heart J* 1995;16:741-51.

2 Aetiology

G Y H Lip, C R Gibbs, D G Beevers

The relative importance of aetiological factors in heart failure is dependent on the nature of the population being studied, as coronary artery disease and hypertension are common causes of heart failure in Western countries, whereas valvar heart disease and nutritional cardiac disease are more common in the developing world. Epidemiological studies are also dependent on the clinical criteria and relevant investigations used for diagnosis, as it remains difficult, for example, to distinguish whether hypertension is the primary cause of heart failure or whether there is also underlying coronary artery disease.

Coronary artery disease and its risk factors

Coronary heart disease is the commonest cause of heart failure in Western countries. In the studies of left ventricular dysfunction (SOLVD) coronary artery disease accounted for almost 75% of the cases of chronic heart failure in male white patients, although in the Framingham heart study, coronary heart disease accounted for only 46% of cases of heart failure in men and 27% of chronic heart failure cases in women. Coronary artery disease and hypertension (either alone or in combination) were implicated as the cause in over 90% of cases of heart failure in the Framingham study.

Recent studies that have allocated aetiology on the basis of non-invasive investigations—such as the Hillingdon heart failure study—have identified coronary artery disease as the primary aetiology in 36% of cases of heart failure. In the Hillingdon study, however, researchers were not able to identify the primary aetiology in 34% of cases; this methodological failing has been addressed in the current Bromley heart failure study, which uses coronary angiography as well as historical and non-invasive findings.

Coronary risk factors, such as smoking and diabetes mellitus, are also risk markers of the development of heart failure. Smoking is an independent and strong risk factor for the development of heart failure in men, although the findings in women are less consistent.

In the prevention arm of SOLVD diabetes was an independent risk factor (about twofold) for mortality, the

---

Causes of heart failure

Coronary artery disease
- Myocardial infarction
- Ischaemia

Hypertension

Cardiomyopathy
- Dilated (congestive)
- Hypertrophic/obstructive
- Restrictive—for example, amyloidosis, sarcoidosis, haemochromatosis
- Obliterative

Valvar and congenital heart disease
- Mitral valve disease
- Aortic valve disease
- Atrial septal defect, ventricular septal defect

Arrhythmias
- Tachycardia
- Bradycardia (complete heart block, the sick sinus syndrome)
- Loss of atrial transport—for example, atrial fibrillation

Alcohol and drugs
- Alcohol
- Cardiac depressant drugs (β blockers, calcium antagonists)

"High output" failure
- Anaemia, thyrotoxicosis, arteriovenous fistulae, Paget's disease

Pericardial disease
- Constrictive pericarditis
- Pericardial effusion

Primary right heart failure
- Pulmonary hypertension—for example, pulmonary embolism, cor pulmonale
- Tricuspid incompetence

Epidemiological studies of aetiology of heart failure. Values are percentages

Aetiology	Teerlink et al (31 studies 1989-90)	Framingham heart study* Men	Framingham heart study* Women	Hillingdon study
Ischaemic	50	59	48	36
Non-ischaemic:	50	41	52	64
Hypertension	4	70	78	14
Idiopathic	18	0	0	0
Valvar	4	22	31	7
Other	10	7	7	10
"Unknown"	13	0	0	34

Because of rounding, totals may not equal 100%.
*Total exceeds 100% as coronary artery disease and hypertension were not considered as mutually exclusive causes.

Relative risks for development of heart failure: 36 year follow up in Framingham heart study

Variable	Age (years) Men 35-64	Men 65-94	Women 35-64	Women 65-94
Serum cholesterol (>6.3 mmol/l)	1.2	0.9	0.7	0.8
Hypertension (>160/95 mm Hg or receiving treatment)	4.0	1.9	3.0	1.9
Glucose intolerance	4.4	2.0	7.7	3.6
Electrocardiographic left ventricular hypertrophy	15.0	4.9	12.8	5.4

development of heart failure, and admission to hospital for heart failure, whereas in the Framingham study diabetes and left ventricular hypertrophy were the most significant risk markers of the development of heart failure. Body weight and a high ratio of total cholesterol concentration to high density lipoprotein cholesterol concentration are also independent risk factors for heart failure. Clearly, these risk factors may increase the risks of heart failure through their effects on coronary artery disease, although diabetes alone may induce important structural and functional changes in the myocardium, which further increase the risk of heart failure.

Hypertension

Hypertension has been associated with an increased risk of heart failure in several epidemiological studies. In the Framingham heart study, hypertension was reported as the cause of heart failure—either alone or in association with other factors—in over 70% of cases, on the basis of non-invasive assessment. Other community and hospital based studies, however, have reported hypertension to be a less common cause of heart failure, and, indeed, the importance of hypertension as a cause of heart failure has been declining in the Framingham cohort since the 1950s. Recent community based studies that have assessed aetiology using clinical criteria and relevant non-invasive investigations have reported hypertension to be the cause of heart failure in 10-20%. However, hypertension is probably a more common cause of heart failure in selected patient groups, including females and black populations (up to a third of cases).

Hypertension predisposes to the development of heart failure via a number of pathological mechanisms, including left ventricular hypertrophy. Left ventricular hypertrophy is associated with left ventricular systolic and diastolic dysfunction and an increased risk of myocardial infarction, and it predisposes to both atrial and ventricular arrhythmias. Electrocardiographic left ventricular hypertrophy is strongly correlated with the development of heart failure, as it is associated with a 14-fold increase in the risk of heart failure in those aged 65 years or under.

Cardiomyopathies

Cardiomyopathies are defined as the diseases of heart muscle that are not secondary to coronary disease, hypertension, or congenital, valvar, or pericardial disease. As primary diseases of heart muscle, cardiomyopathies are less common causes of heart failure, but awareness of their existence is necessary to make a diagnosis. Cardiomyopathies are separated into four functional categories: dilated (congestive), hypertrophic, restrictive, and obliterative. These groups can include rare, specific heart muscle diseases (such as haemochromatosis (iron overload) and metabolic and endocrine disease), in which cardiac involvement occurs as part of a systemic disorder. Dilated cardiomyopathy is a more common cause of heart failure than hypertrophic and restrictive cardiomyopathies; obliterative cardiomyopathy is essentially limited to developing countries.

Dilated cardiomyopathy

Dilated cardiomyopathy describes heart muscle disease in which the predominant abnormality is dilatation of the left ventricle, with or without right ventricular dilatation. Myocardial cells are also hypertrophied, with increased variation in size and increased extracellular fibrosis. Family studies have reported

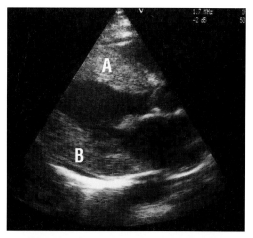

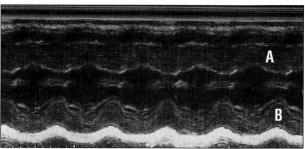

Two dimensional echocardiogram (top) and M mode echocardiogram (bottom) showing left ventricular hypertrophy. A=interventricular septum; B=posterior left ventricular wall

Effective blood pressure lowering in patients with hypertension reduces the risk of heart failure; an overview of trials has estimated that effective antihypertensive treatment reduces the age standardised incidence of heart failure by up to 50%

Causes of dilated cardiomyopathy

Familial

Infectious
- Viral (coxsackie B, cytomegalovirus, HIV)
- Rickettsia
- Bacteria (diphtheria)
- Mycobacteria
- Fungus
- Parasites (Chagas' disease, toxoplasmosis)
- Alcohol
- Cardiotoxic drugs (adriamycin, doxorubicin, zidovudine)
- Cocaine
- Metals (cobalt, mercury, lead)
- Nutritional disease (beriberi, kwashiorkor, pellagra)
- Endocrine disease (myxoedema, thyrotoxicosis, acromegaly, phaeochromocytoma)

Pregnancy

Collagen disease
- Connective tissue diseases (systemic lupus erythematosus, scleroderma, polyarteritis nodosa)

Neuromuscular
- Duchenne muscular dystrophy, myotonic dystrophy

Idiopathic

that up to a quarter of cases of dilated cardiomyopathy have a familial basis. Viral myocarditis is a recognised cause; connective tissue diseases such as systemic lupus erythematosus, the Churg-Strauss syndrome, and polyarteritis nodosa are rarer causes. Idiopathic dilated cardiomyopathy is a diagnosis of exclusion. Coronary angiography will exclude coronary disease, and an endomyocardial biopsy is required to exclude underlying myocarditis or an infiltrative disease.

Dilatation can be associated with the development of atrial and ventricular arrhythmias, and dilatation of the ventricles leads to "functional" mitral and tricuspid valve regurgitation.

Hypertrophic cardiomyopathy

Hypertrophic cardiomyopathy has a familial inheritance (autosomal dominant), although sporadic cases may occur. It is characterised by abnormalities of the myocardial fibres, and in its classic form involves asymmetrical septal hypertrophy, which may be associated with aortic outflow obstruction (hypertrophic obstructive cardiomyopathy).

Nevertheless, other forms of hypertrophic cardiomyopathy exist—apical hypertrophy (especially in Japan) and symmetrical left ventricular hypertrophy (where the echocardiographic distinction between this and hypertensive heart disease may be unclear). These abnormalities lead to poor left ventricular compliance, with high end diastolic pressures, and there is a common association with atrial and ventricular arrhythmias, the latter leading to sudden cardiac death. Mitral regurgitation may contribute to the heart failure in these patients.

Restrictive and obliterative cardiomyopathies

Restrictive cardiomyopathy is characterised by a stiff and poorly compliant ventricle, which is not substantially enlarged, and this is associated with abnormalities of diastolic function (relaxation) that limit ventricular filling. Amyloidosis and other infiltrative diseases, including sarcoidosis and haemochromatosis, can cause a restrictive syndrome. Endomyocardial fibrosis is also a cause of restrictive cardiomyopathy, although it is a rare cause of heart failure in Western countries. Endocardial fibrosis of the inflow tract of one or both ventricles, including the subvalvar regions, results in restriction of diastolic filling and cavity obliteration.

Valvar disease

Rheumatic heart disease may have declined in certain parts of the world, but it still represents an important cause of heart failure in India and other developing nations. In the Framingham study rheumatic heart disease accounted for heart failure in 2% of men and 3% of women, although the overall incidence of valvar disease has been steadily decreasing in the Framingham cohort over the past 30 years.

Mitral regurgitation and aortic stenosis are the most common causes of heart failure, secondary to valvar disease. Mitral regurgitation (and aortic regurgitation) leads to volume overload (increased preload), in contrast with aortic stenosis, which leads to pressure overload (increased afterload). The progression of heart failure in patients with valvar disease is dependent on the nature and extent of the valvar disease. In aortic stenosis heart failure develops at a relatively late stage and, without valve replacement, it is associated with a poor prognosis. In contrast, patients with chronic mitral (or aortic) regurgitation generally decline in a slower and more progressive manner.

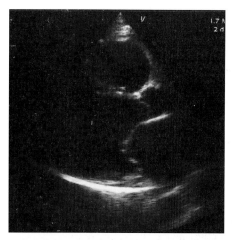

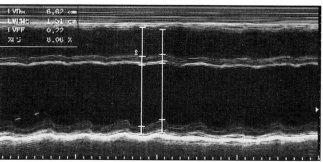

Two dimensional (long axis parasternal view) echocardiogram (top) and M mode echocardiogram (bottom) showing severely impaired left ventricular function in dilated cardiomyopathy

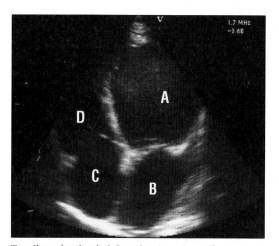

Two dimensional, apical, four chamber echocardiogram showing dilated cardiomyopathy. A=left ventricle; B=left atrium; C=right atrium; D=right ventricle

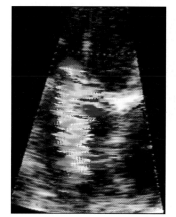
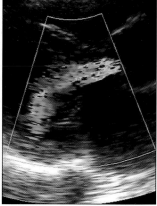

Colour Doppler echocardiograms showing mitral regurgitation (left) and aortic regurgitation (right)

Arrhythmias

Cardiac arrhythmias are more common in patients with heart failure and associated structural heart disease, including hypertensive patients with left ventricular hypertrophy. Atrial fibrillation and heart failure often coexist, and this has been confirmed in large scale trials and smaller hospital based studies. In the Hillingdon heart failure study 30% of patients presenting for the first time with heart failure had atrial fibrillation, and over 60% of patients admitted urgently with atrial fibrillation to a Glasgow hospital had echocardiographic evidence of impaired left ventricular function.

Atrial fibrillation in patients with heart failure has been associated with increased mortality in some studies, although the vasodilator heart failure trial (V-HeFT) failed to show an increase in major morbidity or mortality for patients with atrial fibrillation. In the stroke prevention in atrial fibrillation (SPAF) study, the presence of concomitant heart failure or left ventricular dysfunction increased the risk of stroke and thromboembolism in patients with atrial fibrillation. Ventricular arrhythmias are also more common in heart failure, leading to a sudden deterioration in some patients; such arrhythmias are a major cause of sudden death in patients with heart failure.

Alcohol and drugs

Alcohol has a direct toxic effect on the heart, which may lead to acute heart failure or heart failure as a result of arrhythmias, commonly atrial fibrillation. Excessive chronic alcohol consumption also leads to dilated cardiomyopathy (alcoholic heart muscle disease). Alcohol is the identifiable cause of chronic heart failure in 2-3% of cases. Rarely, alcohol misuse may be associated with general nutritional deficiency and thiamine deficiency (beriberi).

Chemotherapeutic agents (for example, doxorubicin) and antiviral drugs (for example, zidovudine) have been implicated in heart failure, through direct toxic effects on the myocardium.

Other causes

Infections may precipitate heart failure as a result of the toxic metabolic effects (relative hypoxia, acid base disturbance) in combination with peripheral vasodilation and tachycardia, leading to increased myocardial oxygen demand. Patients with chronic heart failure, like patients with most chronic illnesses, are particularly susceptible to viral and bacterial respiratory infections. "High output" heart failure is most often seen in patients with severe anaemia, although thyrotoxicosis may also be a precipitating cause in these patients. Myxoedema may present with heart failure as a result of myocardial involvement or secondary to a pericardial effusion.

The table of epidemiological studies of the aetiology of heart failure is adapted and reproduced with permission from Cowie MR et al (*Eur Heart J* 1997;18:208-25). The table showing relative risks for development of heart failure (36 year follow up) is adapted and reproduced with permission from Kannel WB et al (*Br Heart J* 1994;72:S3-9).

Arrhythmias and heart failure: mechanisms

Tachycardias
- Reduce diastolic ventricular filling time
- Increase myocardial workload and myocardial oxygen demand, precipitating ischaemia
- If they are chronic, with poor rate control, they may lead to ventricular dilatation and impaired ventricular function ("tachycardia induced cardiomyopathy")

Bradycardias
- Compensatory increase in stroke volume is limited in the presence of structural heart disease, and cardiac output is reduced

Abnormal atrial and ventricular contraction
- Loss of atrial systole leads to the absence of active ventricular filling, which in turn lowers cardiac output and raises atrial pressure—for example, atrial fibrillation
- Dissociation of atrial and ventricular activity impairs diastolic ventricular filling, particularly in the presence of a tachycardia—for example, ventricular tachycardia

---

Prevalence (%) of atrial fibrillation in major heart failure trials

Trial	NYHA class*	Prevalence of atrial fibrillation
SOLVD	I–III	6
V-HeFT I	II–III	15
V-HeFT II	II–III	15
CONSENSUS	III–IV	50

CONSENSUS = cooperative north Scandinavian enalapril survival study.
*Classification of the New York Heart Association.

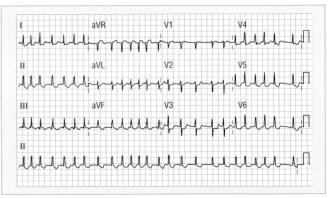

Electrocardiogram showing atrial fibrillation with a rapid ventricular response

---

Key references
- Cowie MR, Wood DA, Coats AJS, Thompson SG, Poole-Wilson PA, Suresh V, et al. Incidence and aetiology of heart failure: a population-based study. *Eur Heart J* 1999;20:421-8.
- Eriksson H, Svardsudd K, Larsson B, Ohlson LO, Tibblin G, Welin L, et al. Risk factors for heart failure in the general population: the study of men born in 1913. *Eur Heart J* 1989;10:647-56.
- Levy D, Larson MG, Vasan RS, Kannel WB, Ho KKL. The progression from hypertension to congestive heart failure. *JAMA* 1996;275:1557-62.
- Oakley C. Aetiology, diagnosis, investigation, and management of cardiomyopathies. *BMJ* 1997;315:1520-4.
- Teerlink JR, Goldhaber SZ, Pfeffer MA. An overview of contemporary etiologies of congestive heart failure. *Am Heart J* 1991;121:1852-3.
- Wheeldon NM, MacDonald TM, Flucker CJ, McKendrick AD, McDevitt DG, Struthers AD. Echocardiography in chronic heart failure in the community. *Q J Med* 1993;86:17-23.

3 Pathophysiology

G Jackson, C R Gibbs, M K Davies, G Y H Lip

Heart failure is a multisystem disorder which is characterised by abnormalities of cardiac, skeletal muscle, and renal function; stimulation of the sympathetic nervous system; and a complex pattern of neurohormonal changes.

Myocardial systolic dysfunction

The primary abnormality in non-valvar heart failure is an impairment in left ventricular function, leading to a fall in cardiac output. The fall in cardiac output leads to activation of several neurohormonal compensatory mechanisms aimed at improving the mechanical environment of the heart. Activation of the sympathetic system, for example, tries to maintain cardiac output with an increase in heart rate, increased myocardial contractility, and peripheral vasoconstriction (increased catecholamines). Activation of the renin-angiotensin-aldosterone system (RAAS) also results in vasoconstriction (angiotensin) and an increase in blood volume, with retention of salt and water (aldosterone). Concentrations of vasopressin and natriuretic peptides increase. Furthermore, there may be progressive cardiac dilatation or alterations in cardiac structure (remodelling), or both.

Neurohormonal activation

Chronic heart failure is associated with neurohormonal activation and alterations in autonomic control. Although these compensatory neurohormonal mechanisms provide valuable support for the heart in normal physiological circumstances, they also have a fundamental role in the development and subsequent progression of chronic heart failure.

Renin-angiotensin-aldosterone system
Stimulation of the renin-angiotensin-aldosterone system leads to increased concentrations of renin, plasma angiotensin II, and aldosterone. Angiotensin II is a potent vasoconstrictor of the renal (efferent arterioles) and systemic circulation, where it stimulates release of noradrenaline from sympathetic nerve terminals, inhibits vagal tone, and promotes the release of aldosterone. This leads to the retention of sodium and water and the increased excretion of potassium. In addition, angiotensin II has important effects on cardiac myocytes and may contribute to the endothelial dysfunction that is observed in chronic heart failure.

Sympathetic nervous system
The sympathetic nervous system is activated in heart failure, via low and high pressure baroreceptors, as an early compensatory mechanism which provides inotropic support and maintains cardiac output. Chronic sympathetic activation, however, has deleterious effects, causing a further deterioration in cardiac function.

The earliest increase in sympathetic activity is detected in the heart, and this seems to precede the increase in sympathetic outflow to skeletal muscle and the kidneys that is present in advanced heart failure. Sustained sympathetic stimulation activates the renin-angiotensin-aldosterone system and other neurohormones, leading to increased venous and arterial tone (and greater preload and afterload respectively), increased

Developments in our understanding of the pathophysiology of heart failure have been essential for recent therapeutic advances in this area

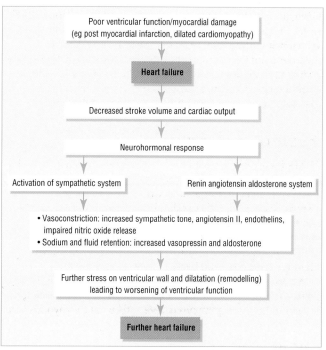

Neurohormonal mechanisms and compensatory mechanisms in heart failure

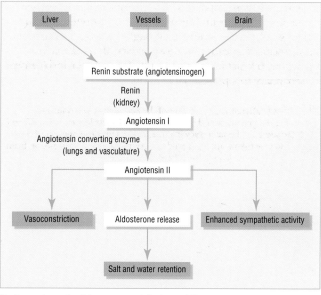

Renin-angiotensin-aldosterone axis in heart failure

plasma noradrenaline concentrations, progressive retention of salt and water, and oedema. Excessive sympathetic activity is also associated with cardiac myocyte apoptosis, hypertrophy, and focal myocardial necrosis.

In the long term, the ability of the myocardium to respond to chronic high concentrations of catecholamines is attenuated by a down regulation in β receptors, although this may be associated with baroreceptor dysfunction and a further increase in sympathetic activity. Indeed, abnormalities of baroreceptor function are well documented in chronic heart failure, along with reduced parasympathetic tone, leading to abnormal autonomic modulation of the sinus node. Moreover, a reduction in heart rate variability has consistently been observed in chronic heart failure, as a result of predominantly sympathetic and reduced vagal modulation of the sinus node, which may be a prognostic marker in patients with chronic heart failure.

Natriuretic peptides

There are three natriuretic peptides, of similar structure, and these exert a wide range of effects on the heart, kidneys, and central nervous system.

Atrial natriuretic peptide (ANP) is released from the atria in response to stretch, leading to natriuresis and vasodilatation. In humans, brain natriuretic peptide (BNP) is also released from the heart, predominantly from the ventricles, and its actions are similar to those of atrial natriuretic peptide. C-type natriuretic peptide is limited to the vascular endothelium and central nervous system and has only limited effects on natriuresis and vasodilatation.

The atrial and brain natriuretic peptides increase in response to volume expansion and pressure overload of the heart and act as physiological antagonists to the effects of angiotensin II on vascular tone, aldosterone secretion, and renal-tubule sodium reabsorption. As the natriuretic peptides are important mediators, with increased circulating concentrations in patients with heart failure, interest has developed in both the diagnostic and prognostic potential of these peptides. Substantial interest has been expressed about the therapeutic potential of natriuretic peptides, particularly with the development of agents that inhibit the enzyme that metabolises atrial natriuretic peptide (neutral endopeptidase), and non-peptide agonists for the A and B receptors.

Antidiuretic hormone (vasopressin)

Antidiuretic hormone concentrations are also increased in severe chronic heart failure. High concentrations of the hormone are particularly common in patients receiving diuretic treatment, and this may contribute to the development of hyponatraemia.

Endothelins

Endothelin is secreted by vascular endothelial cells and is a potent vasoconstrictor peptide that has pronounced vasoconstrictor effects on the renal vasculature, promoting the retention of sodium. Importantly, the plasma concentration of endothelin-1 is of prognostic significance and is increased in proportion to the symptomatic and haemodynamic severity of heart failure. Endothelin concentration is also correlated with indices of severity such as the pulmonary artery capillary wedge pressure, need for admission to hospital, and death.

In view of the vasoconstrictor properties of endothelin, interest has developed in endothelin receptor antagonists as cardioprotective agents which inhibit endothelin mediated vascular and myocardial remodelling.

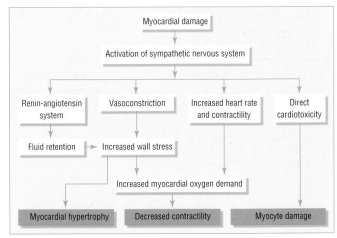

Sympathetic activation in chronic heart failure

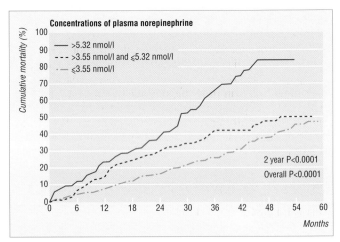

Norepinephrine concentrations and prognosis in chronic heart failure

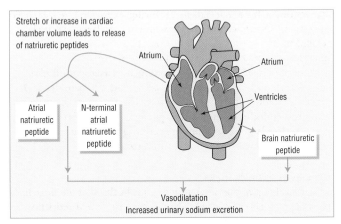

Effects of natriuretic peptides

Other hormonal mechanisms in chronic heart failure

- The arachidonic acid cascade leads to increased concentrations of prostaglandins (prostaglandin E_2 and prostaglandin I_2), which protect the glomerular microcirculation during renal vasoconstriction and maintain glomerular filtration by dilating afferent glomerular arterioles
- The kallikrein kinin system forms bradykinin, resulting in both natriuresis and vasodilatation, and stimulates the production of prostaglandins
- Circulating concentrations of the cytokine tumour necrosis factor (αTNF) are increased in cachectic patients with chronic heart failure. αTNF has also been implicated in the development of endothelial abnormalities in patients with chronic heart failure

Patterns of neurohormonal activation and prognosis

Asymptomatic left ventricular dysfunction

Plasma norepinephrine concentrations increase early in the development of left ventricular dysfunction, and plasma renin activity usually increases in patients receiving diuretic treatment. Norepinephrine concentration in asymptomatic left ventricular dysfunction is a strong and independent predictor of the development of symptomatic chronic heart failure and long term mortality. Plasma concentrations of N-terminal proatrial natriuretic peptide and brain natriuretic peptide also seem to be good indicators of asymptomatic left ventricular dysfunction and may be useful in the future as an objective blood test in these patients.

Congestive heart failure

In severe untreated chronic heart failure, concentrations of renin, angiotensin II, aldosterone, noradrenaline, and atrial natriuretic peptide are all increased. Plasma concentrations of various neuroendocrine markers correlate with both the severity of heart failure and the long term prognosis. For example, raised plasma concentrations of N-terminal and C-terminal atrial natriuretic peptide and of brain natriuretic peptide are independent predictors of mortality in patients with chronic heart failure. Patients with congestive heart failure and raised plasma noradrenaline concentrations also have a worse prognosis.

Other non-cardiac abnormalities in chronic heart failure

Vasculature

The vascular endothelium has an important role in the regulation of vascular tone, releasing relaxing and contracting factors under basal conditions or during exercise. The increased peripheral resistance in patients with chronic heart failure is related to the alterations in autonomic control, including heightened sympathetic tone, activation of the renin-angiotensin-aldosterone system, increased endothelin concentrations, and impaired release of endothelium derived relaxing factor (or nitric oxide). There is emerging evidence that impaired endothelial function in chronic heart failure may be improved with exercise training and drug treatment, such as angiotensin converting enzyme inhibitors.

Skeletal muscle changes

Considerable peripheral changes occur in the skeletal muscle of patients with chronic heart failure. These include a reduction in muscle mass and abnormalities in muscle structure, metabolism, and function. There is also reduced blood flow to active skeletal muscle, which is related to vasoconstriction and the loss in muscle mass. All these abnormalities in skeletal muscles, including respiratory muscles, contribute to the symptoms of fatigue, lethargy, and exercise intolerance that occur in chronic heart failure.

Diastolic dysfunction

Diastolic dysfunction results from impaired myocardial relaxation, with increased stiffness in the ventricular wall and reduced left ventricular compliance, leading to impairment of diastolic ventricular filling. Infiltrations, such as amyloid heart disease, are the best examples, although coronary artery

After myocardial infarction

● Plasma noradrenaline is of prognostic value in patients early after myocardial infarction, predicting subsequent changes in left ventricular volume
● Natriuretic peptides have also been shown to predict outcome after myocardial infarction, although it is not clear whether the predictive value is additive to measurements of ventricular function

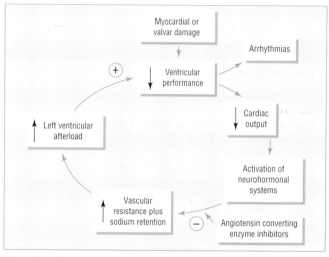

Effect of angiotensin converting enzyme inhibitors in heart failure

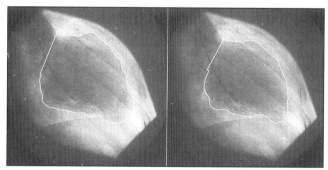

Contrast left ventriculogram in patient with poor systolic function (diastolic (left) and systolic (right) views)

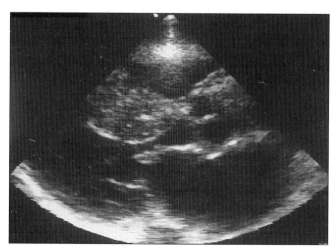

Two dimensional echocardiogram in patient with hypertrophic cardiomyopathy showing asymmetrical septal hypertrophy

disease, hypertension (with left ventricular hypertrophy), and hypertrophic cardiomyopathy are more common causes.

The incidence and contribution of diastolic dysfunction remains controversial, although it has been estimated that 30-40% of patients with heart failure have normal ventricular systolic contraction. Indices of diastolic dysfunction can be obtained non-invasively with Doppler echocardiography or invasively with cardiac catheterisation and measurement of left ventricular pressure changes. There is no agreement as to the most accurate index of left ventricular diastolic dysfunction, but the Doppler mitral inflow velocity profile is probably the most widely used.

Although pure forms exist, in most patients with heart failure both systolic and diastolic dysfunction can be present. Knowing about diastolic dysfunction, however, has little effect on management of most patients with chronic heart failure, as there are still many uncertainties over its measurement and optimal management strategies.

Myocardial remodelling, hibernation, and stunning

After extensive myocardial infarction, cardiac contractility is frequently impaired and neurohormonal activation leads to regional eccentric and concentric hypertrophy of the non-infarcted segment, with expansion (regional thinning and dilatation) of the infarct zone. This is known as remodelling. Particular risk factors for this development of progressive ventricular dilatation after a myocardial infarction include a large infarct, anterior infarctions, occlusion (or non-reperfusion) of the artery related to the infarct, and hypertension.

Myocardial dysfunction may also occur in response to "stunning" (postischaemic dysfunction), which describes delayed recovery of myocardial function despite restoration of coronary blood flow, in the absence of irreversible damage. This is in contrast to "hibernating" myocardium, which describes persistent myocardial dysfunction at rest, secondary to reduced myocardial perfusion, although cardiac myocytes remain viable and myocardial contraction may improve with revascularisation.

When stunning or hibernation occurs, viable myocardium retains responsiveness to inotropic stimulation, which can then be identified by resting and stress echocardiography, thallium scintigraphy and positron emission tomography. Revascularisation may improve the overall left ventricular function with potential beneficial effects on symptoms and prognosis.

Key references

- Grossman W. Diastolic dysfunction in congestive heart failure. *N Engl J Med* 1991;325:1557-64.
- Love MP, McMurray JJV. Endothelin in heart failure: a promising therapeutic target. *Heart* 1997;77:93-4.
- McDonagh TA, Robb SD, Murdoch DR, Morton JJ, Ford I, Morrison CE, et al. Biochemical detection of left ventricular systolic dysfunction. *Lancet* 1998;351:9-13.
- Rahimtoola SH. The hibernating myocardium. *Am Heart J* 1989;117:211-21.
- Wilkins MR, Redondo J, Brown LA. The natriuretic-peptide family. *Lancet* 1997;349:1307-10.
- Packer M. The neurohormonal hypothesis: a theory to explain the mechanisms of disease progression in heart failure. *J Am Coll Cardiol* 1992;20:248-54.

The graph showing mortality curves is adapted from Cohn et al (*N Engl J Med* 1984;311:819-23); the diagram of the process of ventricular remodelling is adapted from McKay et al (*Circulation* 1986;74:693-702).

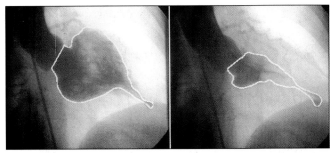

Contrast left ventriculogram in patient with hypertrophic cardiomyopathy (diastolic (left) and systolic (right) views)

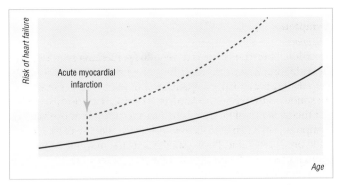

Risk of heart failure and relation with age and history of myocardial infarction

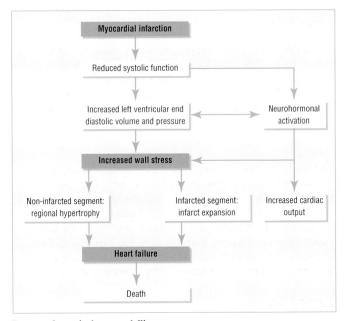

Process of ventricular remodelling

4 Clinical features and complications

R D S Watson, C R Gibbs, G Y H Lip

Clinical features

Patients with heart failure present with a variety of symptoms, most of which are non-specific. The common symptoms of congestive heart failure include fatigue, dyspnoea, swollen ankles, and exercise intolerance, or symptoms that relate to the underlying cause. The accuracy of diagnosis by presenting clinical features alone, however, is often inadequate, particularly in women and elderly or obese patients.

Symptoms

Dyspnoea

Exertional breathlessness is a frequent presenting symptom in heart failure, although it is a common symptom in the general population, particularly in patients with pulmonary disease. Dyspnoea is therefore moderately sensitive, but poorly specific, for the presence of heart failure. Orthopnoea is a more specific symptom, although it has a low sensitivity and therefore has little predictive value. Paroxysmal nocturnal dyspnoea results from increased left ventricular filling pressures (due to nocturnal fluid redistribution and enhanced renal reabsorption) and therefore has a greater sensitivity and predictive value. Nocturnal ischaemic chest pain may also be a manifestation of heart failure, so left ventricular systolic dysfunction should be excluded in patients with recurrent nocturnal angina.

Fatigue and lethargy

Fatigue and lethargy in chronic heart failure are, in part, related to abnormalities in skeletal muscle, with premature muscle lactate release, impaired muscle blood flow, deficient endothelial function, and abnormalities in skeletal muscle structure and function. Reduced cerebral blood flow, when accompanied by abnormal sleep patterns, may occasionally lead to somnolence and confusion in severe chronic heart failure.

Oedema

Swelling of ankles and feet is another common presenting feature, although there are numerous non-cardiac causes of this symptom. Right heart failure may manifest as oedema, right hypochondrial pain (liver distension), abdominal swelling (ascites), loss of appetite, and, rarely, malabsorption (bowel oedema). An increase in weight may be associated with fluid retention, although cardiac cachexia and weight loss are important markers of disease severity in some patients.

Physical signs

Physical examination has serious limitations as many patients, particularly those with less severe heart failure, have few abnormal signs. In addition, some physical signs are difficult to interpret and, if present, may occasionally be related to causes other than heart failure.

Oedema and a tachycardia, for example, are too insensitive to have any useful predictive value, and although pulmonary crepitations may have a high diagnostic specificity they have a low sensitivity and predictive value. Indeed, the commonest cause of lower limb oedema in elderly people is immobility, and pulmonary crepitations may reflect poor ventilation with infection, or pulmonary fibrosis, rather than heart failure. Jugular venous distension has a high specificity in diagnosing heart failure in patients who are known to have cardiac disease,

---

Symptoms and signs in heart failure

Symptoms
Dyspnoea
Orthopnoea
Paroxysmal nocturnal dyspnoea
Reduced exercise tolerance, lethargy, fatigue
Nocturnal cough
Wheeze
Ankle swelling
Anorexia

Signs
Cachexia and muscle wasting
Tachycardia
Pulsus alternans
Elevated jugular venous pressure
Displaced apex beat
Right ventricular heave
Crepitations or wheeze
Third heart sound
Oedema
Hepatomegaly (tender)
Ascites

Common causes of lower limb oedema

- Gravitational disorder—for example, immobility
- Congestive heart failure
- Venous thrombosis or obstruction, varicose veins
- Hypoproteinaemia—for example, nephrotic syndrome, liver disease
- Lymphatic obstruction

Sensitivity, specificity, and predictive value of symptoms, signs, and chest *x* ray findings for presence of heart failure (ejection fraction <40%) in 1306 patients with coronary artery disease undergoing cardiac catheterisation

Clinical features	Sensitivity (%)	Specificity (%)	Positive predictive value (%)
History:			
Shortness of breath	66	52	23
Orthopnoea	21	81	2
Paroxysmal nocturnal dyspnoea	33	76	26
History of oedema	23	80	22
Examination:			
Tachycardia (>100 beats/min)	7	99	6
Crepitations	13	91	27
Oedema (on examination)	10	93	3
Gallop (S3)	31	95	61
Neck vein distension	10	97	2
Chest *x* ray examination:			
Cardiomegaly	62	67	32

although some patients, even with documented heart failure, do not have an elevated venous pressure. The presence of a displaced apex beat in a patient with a history of myocardial infarction has a high positive predictive value. A third heart sound has a relatively high specificity, although its universal value is limited by a high interobserver variability, with interobserver agreement of less than 50% in non-specialists.

In patients with pre-existing chronic heart failure, other clinical features may be evident that point towards precipitating causes of acute heart failure or deteriorating heart failure. Common factors that may be obvious on clinical assessment and are associated with relapses in congestive heart failure include infections, arrhythmias, continued or recurrent myocardial ischaemia, and anaemia.

Clinical diagnosis and clinical scoring systems

Several epidemiological studies, including the Framingham heart study, have used clinical scoring systems to define heart failure, although the use of these systems is not recommended for routine clinical practice.

In a patient with appropriate symptoms and a number of physical signs, including a displaced apex beat, elevated venous pressure, oedema, and a third heart sound, the clinical diagnosis of heart failure may be made with some confidence. However, the clinical suspicion of heart failure should also be confirmed with objective investigations and the demonstration of cardiac dysfunction at rest. It is important to note that, in some patients, exercise-induced myocardial ischaemia may lead to a rise in ventricular filling pressures and a fall in cardiac output, leading to symptoms of heart failure during exertion.

Classification

Symptoms and exercise capacity are used to classify the severity of heart failure and monitor the response to treatment. The classification of the New York Heart Association (NYHA) is used widely, although outcome in heart failure is best determined not only by symptoms (NYHA class) but also by echocardiographic criteria. As the disease is progressive, the importance of early treatment, in an attempt to prevent progression to more severe disease, cannot be overemphasised.

Complications

Arrhythmias

Atrial fibrillation

Atrial fibrillation is present in about a third (range 10-50%) of patients with chronic heart failure and may represent either a cause or a consequence of heart failure. The onset of atrial fibrillation with a rapid ventricular response may precipitate overt heart failure, particularly in patients with pre-existing ventricular dysfunction. Predisposing causes should be considered, including mitral valve disease, thyrotoxicosis, and sinus node disease. Importantly, sinus node disease may be associated with bradycardias, which might be exacerbated by antiarrhythmic treatment.

Atrial fibrillation that occurs with severe left ventricular dysfunction following myocardial infarction is associated with a poor prognosis. In addition, patients with heart failure and atrial fibrillation are at particularly high risk of stroke and other thromboembolic complications.

Ventricular arrhythmias

Malignant ventricular arrhythmias are common in end stage heart failure. For example, sustained monomorphic ventricular

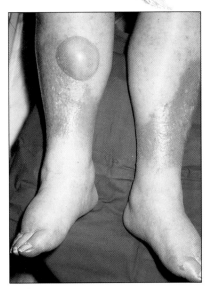

Gross oedema of ankles, including bullae with serous exudate

Precipitating causes of heart failure

- Arrhythmias, especially atrial fibrillation
- Infections (especially pneumonia)
- Acute myocardial infarction
- Angina pectoris or recurrent myocardial ischaemia
- Anaemia
- Alcohol excess
- Iatrogenic cause—for example, postoperative fluid replacement or administration of steroids or non-steroidal anti-inflammatory drugs
- Poor drug compliance, especially in antihypertensive treatment
- Thyroid disorders—for example, thyrotoxicosis
- Pulmonary embolism
- Pregnancy

European Society of Cardiology's guidelines for diagnosis of heart failure

Essential features
Symptoms of heart failure (for example, breathlessness, fatigue, ankle swelling)
and
Objective evidence of cardiac dysfunction (at rest)

Non-essential features
Response to treatment directed towards heart failure (in cases where the diagnosis is in doubt)

NYHA classification of heart failure

Class I: asymptomatic
No limitation in physical activity despite presence of heart disease. This can be suspected only if there is a history of heart disease which is confirmed by investigations—for example, echocardiography

Class II: mild
Slight limitation in physical activity. More strenuous activity causes shortness of breath—for example, walking on steep inclines and several flights of steps. Patients in this group can continue to have an almost normal lifestyle and employment

Class III: moderate
More marked limitation of activity which interferes with work. Walking on the flat produces symptoms

Class IV: severe
Unable to carry out any physical activity without symptoms. Patients are breathless at rest and mostly housebound

tachycardia occurs in up to 10% of patients with advanced heart failure who are referred for cardiac transplantation. In patients with ischaemic heart disease these arrhythmias often have re-entrant mechanisms in scarred myocardial tissue. An episode of sustained ventricular tachycardia indicates a high risk for recurrent ventricular arrhythmias and sudden cardiac death.

Sustained polymorphic ventricular tachycardia and torsades de pointes are more likely to occur in the presence of precipitating or aggravating factors, including electrolyte disturbance (for example, hypokalaemia or hyperkalaemia, hypomagnesaemia), prolonged QT interval, digoxin toxicity, drugs causing electrical instability (for example, antiarrhythmic drugs, antidepressants), and continued or recurrent myocardial ischaemia. β Blockers are useful for treating arrhythmias, and these agents (for example, bisoprolol, metoprolol, carvedilol) are likely to be increasingly used as a treatment option in patients with heart failure.

Stroke and thromboembolism

Congestive heart failure predisposes to stroke and thromboembolism, with an overall estimated annual incidence of approximately 2%. Factors contributing to the increased thromboembolic risk in patients with heart failure include low cardiac output (with relative stasis of blood in dilated cardiac chambers), regional wall motion abnormalities (including formation of a left ventricular aneurysm), and associated atrial fibrillation. Although the prevalence of atrial fibrillation in some of the earlier observational studies was between 12% and 36%—which may have accounted for some of the thromboembolic events—patients with chronic heart failure who remain in sinus rhythm are also at an increased risk of stroke and venous thromboembolism. Patients with heart failure and chronic venous insufficiency may also be immobile, and this contributes to their increased risk of thrombosis, including deep venous thrombosis and pulmonary embolism.

Recent observational data from the studies of left ventricular dysfunction (SOLVD) and vasodilator heart failure trials (V-HeFT) indicate that mild to moderate heart failure is associated with an annual risk of stroke of about 1.5% (compared with a risk of less than 0.5% in those without heart failure), rising to 4% in patients with severe heart failure. In addition, the survival and ventricular enlargement (SAVE) study recently reported an inverse relation between risk of stroke and left ventricular ejection fraction, with an 18% increase in risk for every 5% reduction in left ventricular ejection fraction; this clearly relates thromboembolism to severe cardiac impairment and the severity of heart failure. As thromboembolic risk seems to be related to left atrial and left ventricular dilatation, echocardiography may have some role in the risk stratification of thromboembolism in patients with chronic heart failure.

Prognosis

Most long term (more than 10 years of follow up) longitudinal studies of heart failure, including the Framingham heart study (1971), were performed before the widespread use of angiotensin converting enzyme inhibitors. In the Framingham study the overall survival at eight years for all NYHA classes was 30%, compared with a one year mortality in classes III and IV of 34% and a one year mortality in class IV of over 60%. The prognosis in patients whose left ventricular dysfunction is asymptomatic is better than that in those whose left ventricular dysfunction is symptomatic. The prognosis in patients with congestive heart failure is dependent on severity, age, and sex, with a poorer prognosis in male patients. In addition, numerous prognostic indices are associated with an adverse prognosis,

---

Predisposing factors for ventricular arrhythmias

- Recurrent or continued coronary ischaemia
- Recurrent myocardial infarction
- Hypokalaemia and hyperkalaemia
- Hypomagnesaemia
- Psychotropic drugs—for example, tricyclic antidepressants
- Digoxin (leading to toxicity)
- Antiarrhythmic drugs that may be cardiodepressant (negative inotropism) and proarrhythmic

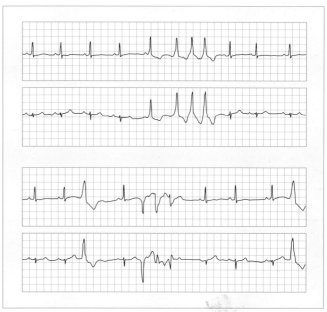

24 Hour Holter tracing showing frequent ventricular extrasystoles

---

Complications of heart failure

Arrhythmias—Atrial fibrillation; ventricular arrhythmias (ventricular tachycardia, ventricular fibrillation); bradyarrhythmias
Thromboembolism—Stroke; peripheral embolism; deep venous thrombosis; pulmonary embolism
Gastrointestinal—Hepatic congestion and hepatic dysfunction; malabsorption
Musculoskeletal—Muscle wasting
Respiratory—Pulmonary congestion; respiratory muscle weakness; pulmonary hypertension (rare)

Morbidity and mortality for all grades of symptomatic chronic heart failure are high, with a 20-30% one year mortality in mild to moderate heart failure and a greater than 50% one year mortality in severe heart failure. These prognostic data refer to patients with systolic heart failure, as the natural course of diastolic dysfunction is less well defined

including NYHA class, left ventricular ejection fraction, and neurohormonal status.

Survival can be prolonged in chronic heart failure that results from systolic dysfunction if angiotensin converting enzyme inhibitors are given. Longitudinal data from the Framingham study and the Mayo Clinic suggest, however, that there is still only a limited improvement in the one year survival rate of patients with newly diagnosed symptomatic chronic heart failure, which remains at 60-70%. In these studies only a minority of patients with congestive heart failure were appropriately treated, with less than 25% of them receiving angiotensin converting enzyme inhibitors, and even among treated patients the dose used was much lower than doses used in the clinical trials.

Some predictors of poor outcome in chronic heart failure

- High NYHA functional class
- Reduced left ventricular ejection fraction
- Low peak oxygen consumption with maximal exercise (% predicted value)
- Third heart sound
- Increased pulmonary artery capillary wedge pressure
- Reduced cardiac index
- Diabetes mellitus
- Reduced sodium concentration
- Raised plasma catecholamine and natriuretic peptide concentrations

---

Cardiac mortality in placebo controlled heart failure trials

| Trial | Patients' characteristics | Ischaemic heart disease (%) | Treatment | Cardiovascular mortality | | Follow up (years) |
				Treatment (%)	Placebo (%)	
CONSENSUS	NYHA IV (cardiomegaly)	73	Enalapril	38	54	1
SOLVD-P	Asymptomatic (EF <35%)	83	Enalapril	13	14	4
SOLVD-T	Symptomatic (EF <35%)	71	Enalapril	31	36	4
SAVE	Postmyocardial infarction (EF <40%)	100	Captopril	17	21	4
V-HeFT I	NYHA II-III (EF <45%)	44	H-ISDN	37	41	5
V-HeFT II	NYHA II-III (EF <45%)	52	Enalapril	28	34*	5
PRAISE	NYHA III-IV (EF <30%)	63	Amlodipine	28	33	1.2

EF ejection fraction. SOLVD-P, SOLVD-T = studies of left ventricular dysfunction prevention arm (P) and treatment arm (T).
H-ISDN = hydralazine and isosorbide dinitrate.
*Treatment with H-ISDN.

Treatment with angiotensin converting enzyme inhibitors prevents or delays the onset of symptomatic heart failure in patients with asymptomatic, or minimally symptomatic, left ventricular systolic dysfunction. The increase in mortality with the development of symptoms suggests that the optimal time for intervention with these agents is well before the onset of substantial left ventricular dysfunction, even in the absence of overt clinical symptoms of heart failure. This benefit has been confirmed in several large, well conducted, postmyocardial infarction studies.

Sudden death

The mode of death in heart failure has been extensively investigated, and progressive heart failure and sudden death seem to occur with equal frequency. Some outstanding questions still remain, however. Although arrhythmias are common in patients with heart failure and are indicators of disease severity, they are not powerful independent predictors of prognosis. Sudden death may be related to ventricular arrhythmias, although asystole is a common terminal event in severe heart failure. It has not been firmly established whether these arrhythmias are primary arrhythmias or whether some are secondary to acute coronary ischaemia or indicate in situ coronary thrombosis. The cause of death is often uncertain, especially as the patient may die of a cardiac arrest outside hospital or while asleep.

Key references

- Doval HC, Nul DR, Grancelli HO, Perrone SV, Bortman GR, Curiel R, et al. Randomised trial of low-dose amiodarone in severe congestive heart failure. *Lancet* 1994;334:493-8.
- Gradman A, Deedwania P, Cody R, Massie B, Packer M, Pitt B, et al. Predictors of total mortality and sudden death in mild to moderate heart failure. *J Am Coll Cardiol* 1989;14:564-70.
- Guidelines for the diagnosis of heart failure. The Task Force on Heart Failure of the European Society of Cardiology. *Eur Heart J* 1995;16:741-51.
- Rodeheffer RJ, Jacobsen SJ, Gersh BJ, Kottke TE, McCann HA, Bailey KR, et al. The incidence and prevalence of congestive heart failure in Rochester, Minnesota. *Mayo Clin Proc* 1993;68:1143-50.
- The SOLVD Investigators. Effect of enalapril on mortality and the development of heart failure in asymptomatic patients with reduced left ventricular ejection fractions. *N Engl J Med* 1992;327:685-91.
- The CONSENSUS Trial Study Group. Effects of enalapril on mortality in severe congestive heart failure: results of the cooperative north Scandinavian enalapril survival study (CONSENSUS). *N Engl J Med* 1987;316:1429-35.

The table on the sensitivity, specificity, and predictive value of symptoms, signs, and chest x ray findings is adapted with permission from Harlan et al (*Ann Intern Med* 1977;86:133-8).

5   Investigation

M K Davies, C R Gibbs, G Y H Lip

Clinical assessment is mandatory before detailed investigations are conducted in patients with suspected heart failure, although specific clinical features are often absent and the condition can be diagnosed accurately only in conjunction with more objective investigation, particularly echocardiography. Although open access echocardiography is now increasingly available, appropriate pre-referral investigations include chest radiography, 12 lead electrocardiography, and renal chemistry.

Chest *x* ray examination

The chest *x* ray examination has an important role in the routine investigation of patients with suspected heart failure, and it may also be useful in monitoring the response to treatment. Cardiac enlargement (cardiothoracic ratio >50%) may be present, but there is a poor correlation between the cardiothoracic ratio and left ventricular function. The presence of cardiomegaly is dependent on both the severity of haemodynamic disturbance and its duration: cardiomegaly is frequently absent, for example, in acute left ventricular failure secondary to acute myocardial infarction, acute valvar regurgitation, or an acquired ventricular septal defect. An increased cardiothoracic ratio may be related to left or right ventricular dilatation, left ventricular hypertrophy, and occasionally a pericardial effusion, particularly if the cardiac silhouette has a globular appearance. Echocardiography is required to distinguish reliably between these different causes, although in decompensated heart failure other radiographic features may be present, such as pulmonary congestion or pulmonary oedema.

In left sided failure, pulmonary venous congestion occurs, initially in the upper zones (referred to as upper lobe diversion or congestion). When the pulmonary venous pressure increases further, usually above 20 mm Hg, fluid may be present in the horizontal fissure and Kerley B lines in the costophrenic angles. In the presence of pulmonary venous pressures above 25 mm Hg, frank pulmonary oedema occurs, with a "bats wing" appearance in the lungs, although this is also dependent on the rate at which the pulmonary oedema has developed. In addition, pleural effusions occur, normally bilaterally, but if they are unilateral the right side is more commonly affected. Nevertheless, it is not possible to distinguish, when viewed in isolation, whether pulmonary congestion is related to cardiac or non-cardiac causes (for example, renal disease, drugs, the respiratory distress syndrome).

Rarely, chest radiography may also show valvar calcification, a left ventricular aneurysm, and the typical pericardial calcification of constrictive pericarditis. Chest radiography may also provide valuable information about non-cardiac causes of dyspnoea.

12 lead electrocardiography

The 12 lead electrocardiographic tracing is abnormal in most patients with heart failure, although it can be normal in up to 10% of cases. Common abnormalities include Q waves, abnormalities in the T wave and ST segment, left ventricular hypertrophy, bundle branch block, and atrial fibrillation. It is a useful screening test as a normal electrocardiographic tracing makes it unlikely that the patient has heart failure secondary to

---

Investigations if heart failure is suspected

Initial investigations
- Chest radiography
- Electrocardiography
- Echocardiography, including Doppler studies
- Haematology tests
- Serum biochemistry, including renal function and glucose concentrations, liver function tests, and thyroid function tests
- Cardiac enzymes (if recent infarction is suspected)

Other investigations
- Radionuclide imaging
- Cardiopulmonary exercise testing
- Cardiac catheterisation
- Myocardial biopsy—for example, in suspected myocarditis

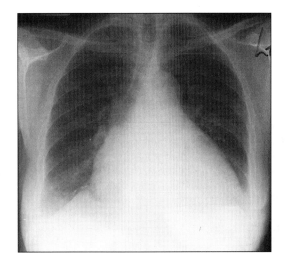

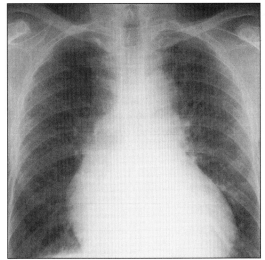

Chest radiographs showing gross cardiomegaly in patient with dilated cardiomyopathy (top); cardiomegaly and pulmonary congestion with fluid in horizontal fissure (bottom)

left ventricular systolic dysfunction, since this test has high sensitivity and a negative predictive value. The combination of a normal chest *x* ray finding and a normal electrocardiographic tracing makes a cardiac cause of dyspnoea very unlikely.

In patients with symptoms (palpitations or dizziness), 24 hour electrocardiographic (Holter) monitoring or a Cardiomemo device will detect paroxysmal arrhythmias or other abnormalities, such as ventricular extrasystoles, sustained or non-sustained ventricular tachycardia, and abnormal atrial rhythms (extrasystoles, supraventricular tachycardia, and paroxysmal atrial fibrillation). Many patients with heart failure, however, show complex ventricular extrasystoles on 24 hour monitoring.

Echocardiography

Echocardiography is the single most useful non-invasive test in the assessment of left ventricular function; ideally it should be conducted in all patients with suspected heart failure. Although clinical assessment, when combined with a chest *x* ray examination and electrocardiography, allows a preliminary diagnosis of heart failure, echocardiography provides an objective assessment of cardiac structure and function. Left ventricular dilatation and impairment of contraction is observed in patients with systolic dysfunction related to ischaemic heart disease (where a regional wall motion abnormality may be detected) or in dilated cardiomyopathy (with global impairment of systolic contraction).

A quantitative measurement can be obtained from calculation of the left ventricular ejection fraction. This is the stroke volume (the difference between the end diastolic and end systolic volumes) expressed as a percentage of the left ventricular end diastolic volume. Measurements, and the assessment of left ventricular function, are less reliable in the presence of atrial fibrillation. The left ventricular ejection fraction has been correlated with outcome and survival in patients with heart failure, although the assessment may be unreliable in patients with regional abnormalities in wall motion. Regional abnormalities can also be quantified into a wall motion index, although in practice the assessment of systolic function is often based on visual assessment and the observer's experience of normal and abnormal contractile function. These abnormalities are described as hypokinetic (reduced systolic contraction), akinetic (no systolic contraction) and dyskinetic (abnormalities of direction or timing of contraction, or both), and refer to universally recognised segments of the left ventricle. Echocardiography may also show other abnormalities, including valvar disease, left ventricular aneurysm, intracardiac thrombus, and pericardial disease.

Mitral incompetence is commonly identified on echocardiography in patients with heart failure, as a result of ventricular and annular dilatation ("functional" mitral incompetence), and this must be distinguished from mitral incompetence related to primary valve disease. Two dimensional echocardiography allows the assessment of valve structure and identifies thickening of cusps, leaflet prolapse, cusp fusion, and calcification. Doppler echocardiography allows the quantitative assessment of flow across valves and the identification of valve stenosis, in addition to the assessment of right ventricular systolic pressures and allowing the indirect diagnosis of pulmonary hypertension. Doppler studies have been used in the assessment of diastolic function, although there is no single reliable echocardiographic measure of diastolic dysfunction. Colour flow Doppler techniques are particularly sensitive in detecting the direction of blood flow and the presence of valve incompetence.

Value of electrocardiography* in identifying heart failure resulting from left ventricular systolic dysfunction

Sensitivity	94%
Specificity	61%
Positive predictive value	35%
Negative predictive value	98%

*Electrocardiographic abnormalities are defined as atrial fibrillation, evidence of previous myocardial infarction, left ventricular hypertrophy, bundle branch block, and left axis deviation.

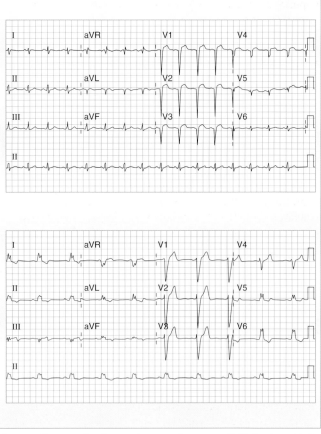

Electrocardiograms showing previous anterior myocardial infarction with Q waves in anteroseptal leads (top) and left bundle branch block (bottom)

Who should have an echocardiogram?

- Almost all patients with symptoms or signs of heart failure
- Symptoms of breathlessness in association with signs of a murmur
- Dyspnoea associated with atrial fibrillation
- Patients at "high risk" for left ventricular dysfunction—for example, those with anterior myocardial infarction, poorly controlled hypertension, or arrhythmias

Echocardiography as a guide to management

- Identification of impaired systolic function for decision on treatment with angiotensin converting enzyme inhibitors
- Identification of diastolic dysfunction or predominantly right ventricular dysfunction
- Identification and assessment of valvar disease
- Assessment of embolic risk (severe left ventricular impairment with mural thrombus)

Advances in echocardiography include the use of contrast agents for visualisation of the walls of the left ventricle in more detail, especially as in about 10% of patients satisfactory images cannot be obtained with standard transthoracic echocardiography. Transoesophageal echocardiography allows the detailed assessment of the atria, valves, pulmonary veins, and any cardiac masses, including thrombi.

The logistic and health economic aspects of large scale screening with echocardiography have been debated, but the development of open access echocardiography heart failure services for general practitioners and the availability of proved treatments for heart failure that improve prognosis, such as angiotensin converting enzyme inhibitors, highlight the importance of an agreed strategy for the echocardiographic assessment of these patients.

Haematology and biochemistry

Routine haematology and biochemistry investigations are recommended to exclude anaemia as a cause of breathlessness and high output heart failure and to exclude important pre-existing metabolic abnormalities. In mild and moderate heart failure, renal function and electrolytes are usually normal. In severe (New York Heart Association, class IV) heart failure, however, as a result of reduced renal perfusion, high dose diuretics, sodium restriction, and activation of the neurohormonal mechanisms (including vasopressin), there is an inability to excrete water, and dilutional hyponatraemia may be present. Hyponatraemia is, therefore, a marker of the severity of chronic heart failure.

A baseline assessment of renal function is important before starting treatment, as the renal blood flow and the glomerular filtration rate fall in severe congestive heart failure. Baseline serum creatinine concentrations are important: increasing creatinine concentrations may occur after the start of treatment, particularly in patients who are receiving angiotensin converting enzyme inhibitors and high doses of diuretics and in patients with renal artery stenosis. Proteinuria is a common finding in severe congestive heart failure.

Hypokalaemia occurs when high dose diuretics are used without potassium supplementation or potassium sparing agents. Hyperkalaemia can also occur in severe congestive heart failure with a low glomerular filtration rate, particularly with the concurrent use of angiotensin converting enzyme inhibitors and potassium sparing diuretics. Both hypokalaemia and hyperkalaemia increase the risk of cardiac arrhythmias; hypomagnesaemia, which is associated with long term diuretic treatment, increases the risk of ventricular arrhythmias. Liver function tests (serum bilirubin, aspartate aminotransferase, and lactate dehydrogenase) are often abnormal in advanced congestive heart failure, as a result of hepatic congestion. Thyroid function tests are also recommended in all patients, in view of the association between thyroid disease and the heart.

Radionuclide methods

Radionuclide imaging—or multigated ventriculography—allows the assessment of the global left and right ventricular function. Images may be obtained in patients where echocardiography is not possible. The most common method labels red cells with technetium-99m and acquires 16 or 32 frames per heart beat by synchronising ("gating") imaging with electrocardiography. This allows the assessment of ejection fraction, systolic filling rate, diastolic emptying rate, and wall motion abnormalities. These variables can be assessed, if necessary, during rest and exercise;

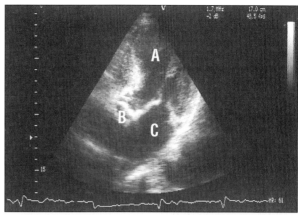

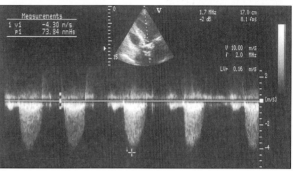

Transthoracic echocardiograms: two dimensional apical view (top) and Doppler studies (bottom) showing severe calcific stenosis, with an estimated aortic gradient of over 70 mm Hg (A=left ventricle, B=aortic valve, and C=left atrium)

Natriuretic peptides

- Biochemical markers are being sought for the diagnosis of congestive heart failure
- Brain natriuretic peptide concentrations correlate with the severity of heart failure and prognosis
- These could, in the future, be used to distinguish between patients in whom heart failure is extremely unlikely and those in whom the probability of heart failure is high
- At present, however, the evidence that blood natriuretic peptide concentrations are valuable in identifying important left ventricular systolic dysfunction is conflicting, and their use in routine practice is still limited
- Further studies are necessary to determine the most convenient and cost effective methods of identifying patients with heart failure and asymptomatic left ventricular dysfunction

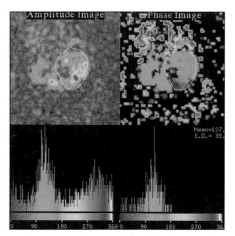

Multigated ventriculography scan in patient with history of extensive myocardial infarction and coronary bypass grafting (left ventricular ejection fraction of 30%)

this method is ideal for the serial reassessment of ejection fraction, but these methods do expose the patient to radiation.

Radionuclide studies are also valuable for assessing myocardial perfusion and the presence or extent of coronary ischaemia, including myocardial stunning and hibernating myocardium.

Angiography, cardiac catheterisation, and myocardial biopsy

Angiography should be considered in patients with recurrent ischaemic chest pain associated with heart failure and in those with evidence of severe reversible ischaemia or hibernating myocardium. Cardiac catheterisation with myocardial biopsy can be valuable in more difficult cases where there is diagnostic doubt—for example, in restrictive and infiltrating cardiomyopathies (amyloid heart disease, sarcoidosis), myocarditis, and pericardial disease. Left ventricular angiography can show global or segmental impairment of function and assess end diastolic pressures, and right heart catheterisation allows an assessment of the right sided pressures (right atrium, right ventricle, and pulmonary arteries) and pulmonary artery capillary wedge pressure, in addition to oxygen saturations.

Pulmonary function tests

Objective measurement of lung function is useful in excluding respiratory causes of breathlessness, although respiratory and cardiac disease commonly coexist. Peak expiratory flow rate and forced expiratory volume in one second are reduced in heart failure, although not as much as in severe chronic obstructive pulmonary disease. In patients with severe breathlessness and wheeze, a peak expiratory flow rate of <200 l/min suggests reversible airways disease, not acute left ventricular failure.

Stress studies use graded physical exercise or pharmacological stress with agents such as adenosine, dipyridamole, and dobutamine. Stress echocardiography is emerging as a useful technique for assessing myocardial reversibility in patients with coronary artery disease

Coronary angiography is essential for accurate assessment of the coronary arteries

Cardiopulmonary exercise testing

- Exercise tolerance is reduced in patients with heart failure, regardless of method of assessment
- Assessment methods include a treadmill test, cycle ergometry, a 6 minute walking test, or pedometry measurements
- Exercise testing is not routinely performed for all patients with congestive heart failure, but it may be valuable in identifying substantial residual ischaemia, thus leading to more detailed investigation
- Respiratory physiological measurements may be made during exercise, and most cardiac transplant centres use data obtained at cardiopulmonary exercise testing to aid the selection of patients for transplantation
- The maximum oxygen consumption is the value at which consumption remains stable despite increasing exercise, and it represents the upper limit of aerobic exercise tolerance
- The maximum oxygen consumption and the carbon dioxide production correlate well with the severity of heart failure
- The maximum oxygen consumption has also been independently related to long term prognosis, especially in patients with severe left ventricular dysfunction

Further reading

- Cheeseman MG, Leech G, Chambers J, Monaghan MJ, Nihoyannopoulos P. Central role of echocardiography in the diagnosis and assessment of heart failure. *Heart* 1998;80(suppl 1):S1-5.
- Dargie HJ, McMurray JVV. Diagnosis and management of heart failure. *BMJ* 1994;308:321-8.
- Schiller NB, Foster E. Analysis of left ventricular systolic function. *Heart* 1996;75(suppl 2):17-26.

The table showing the value of electrocardiography is adapted from Davie et al (*BMJ* 1996;312:222). The table of assessments for the investigation and diagnosis of heart failure is adapted with permission from the Task Force on Heart Failure of the European Society of Cardiology (*Eur Heart J* 1995;16:741-51).

Assessments for the investigation and diagnosis of heart failure

Assessments	Diagnosis of heart failure			Suggests alternative or additional disease
	Necessary	Supports	Opposes	
Symptoms of heart failure	+ +		+ + (if absent)	
Signs of heart failure		+ +	+ (if absent)	
Response to treatment		+ +	+ + (if absent)	
Electrocardiography			+ + (if normal)	
Chest radiography (cardiomegaly or congestion)		+ +	+ (if normal)	Pulmonary
Echocardiography (cardiac dysfunction)	+ +		+ + (if absent)	
Haematology				Anaemia
Biochemistry (renal, liver function, and thyroid function tests)				Renal, liver, thyroid
Urine analysis				Renal
Pulmonary function tests				Pulmonary

+ + = Great importance; + = some importance.

6 Non-drug management

C R Gibbs, G Jackson, G Y H Lip

Approaches to the management of heart failure can be both non-pharmacological and pharmacological; each approach complements the other. This article will discuss non-pharmacological management.

Counselling and education of patients

Effective counselling and education of patients, and of the relatives or carers, is important and may enhance long term adherence to management strategies. Simple explanations about the symptoms and signs of heart failure, including details on drug and other treatment strategies, are valuable. Emphasis should be placed on self help strategies for each patient; these should include information on the need to adhere to drug treatment. Some patients can be instructed how to monitor their weight at home on a daily basis and how to adjust the dose of diuretics as advised; sudden weight increases (>2 kg in 1-3 days), for example, should alert a patient to alter his or her treatment or seek advice.

Lifestyle measures

Urging patients to alter their lifestyle is important in the management of chronic heart failure. Social activities should be encouraged, however, and care should be taken to ensure that patients avoid social isolation. If possible, patients should continue their regular work, with adaptations to accommodate a reduced physical capacity where appropriate.

Contraceptive advice

Advice on contraception should be offered to women of childbearing potential, particularly those patients with advanced heart failure (class III-IV in the New York Heart Association's classification), in whom the risk of maternal morbidity and mortality is high with pregnancy and childbirth. Current hormonal contraceptive methods are much safer than in the past: low dose oestrogen and third generation progestogen derivatives are associated with a relatively low thromboembolic risk.

Smoking

Cigarette smoking should be strongly discouraged in patients with heart failure. In addition to the well established adverse effects on coronary disease, which is the underlying cause in a substantial proportion of patients, smoking has adverse haemodynamic effects in patients with congestive heart failure. For example, smoking tends to reduce cardiac output, especially in patients with a history of myocardial infarction.

Other adverse haemodynamic effects include an increase in heart rate and systemic blood pressure (double product) and mild increases in pulmonary artery pressure, ventricular filling pressures, and total systemic and pulmonary vascular resistance.

The peripheral vasoconstriction may contribute to the observed mild reduction in stroke volume, and thus smoking increases oxygen demand and also decreases myocardial oxygen supply owing to reduced diastolic filling time (with faster heart rates) and increased carboxyhaemoglobin concentrations.

Non-pharmacological measures for the management of heart failure

- Compliance—give careful advice about disease, treatment, and self help strategies
- Diet—ensure adequate general nutrition and, in obese patients, weight reduction
- Salt—advise patients to avoid high salt content foods and not to add salt (particularly in severe cases of congestive heart failure)
- Fluid—urge overloaded patients and those with severe congestive heart failure to restrict their fluid intake
- Alcohol—advise moderate alcohol consumption (abstinence in alcohol related cardiomyopathy)
- Smoking—avoid smoking (adverse effects on coronary disease, adverse haemodynamic effects)
- Exercise—regular exercise should be encouraged
- Vaccination—patients should consider influenza and pneumococcal vaccinations

---

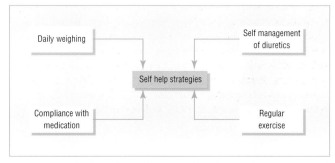

Self help strategies for patients with heart failure

Intrauterine devices are a suitable form of contraception, although these may be a problem in patients with primary valvar disease, in view of the risks of infection and risks associated with oral anticoagulation

---

Menopausal women with heart failure

- Observational data indicate that hormone replacement therapy reduces the risk of coronary events in postmenopausal women
- However, there is limited prospective evidence to advise the use of such therapy in postmenopausal women with heart failure
- Nevertheless, there may be an increased risk of venous thrombosis in postmenopausal women taking hormone replacement therapy, which may exacerbate the risk associated with heart failure

Alcohol

In general, alcohol consumption should be restricted to moderate levels, given the myocardial depressant properties of alcohol. In addition to the direct toxic effects of alcohol on the myocardium, a high alcohol intake predisposes to arrhythmias (especially atrial fibrillation) and hypertension and may lead to important alterations in fluid balance. The prognosis in alcohol induced cardiomyopathy is poor if consumption continues, and abstinence should be advised. Abstinence can result in marked improvements, with echocardiographic studies showing substantial clinical benefit and improvements in left ventricular function. Resumed alcohol consumption may subsequently lead to acute or worsening heart failure.

Immunisation and antiobiotic prophylaxis

Chronic heart failure predisposes to and can be exacerbated by pulmonary infection, and influenza and pneumococcal vaccinations should therefore be considered in all patients with heart failure. Antibiotic prophylaxis, for dental and other surgical procedures, is mandatory in patients with primary valve disease and prosthetic heart valves.

Diet and nutrition

Although controlled trials offer only limited information on diet and nutritional measures, such measures are as important in heart failure, as in any other chronic illness, to ensure adequate and appropriate nutritional balance. Poor nutrition may contribute to cardiac cachexia, although malnutrition is not limited to patients with obvious weight loss and muscle wasting.

Patients with chronic heart failure are at an increased risk from malnutrition owing to (a) a decreased intake resulting from a poor appetite, which may be related to drug treatment (for example, aspirin, digoxin), metabolic disturbance (for example, hyponatraemia or renal failure), or hepatic congestion; (b) malabsorption, particularly in patients with severe heart failure; and (c) increased nutritional requirements, with patients who have congestive heart failure having an increase of up to 20% in basal metabolic rate. These factors may contribute to a net catabolic state where lean muscle mass is reduced, leading to an increase in symptoms and reduced exercise capacity. Indeed, cardiac cachexia is an independent risk factor for mortality in patients with chronic heart failure. A formal nutritional assessment should thus be considered in those patients who appear to have a poor nutritional state.

Weight loss in obese patients should be encouraged as excess body mass increases cardiac workload during exercise. Weight reduction in obese patients to within 10% of the optimal body weight should be encouraged.

Salt restriction

No randomised studies have addressed the role of salt restriction in congestive heart failure. Nevertheless restriction to about 2 g of sodium a day may be useful as an adjunct to treatment with high dose diuretics, particularly if the condition is advanced.

In general, patients should be advised that they should avoid foods that are rich in salt and not to add salt to their food at the table.

Fluid intake

Fluid restriction (1.5-2 litres daily) should be considered in patients with severe symptoms, those requiring high dose diuretics, and those with a tendency towards excessive fluid intake. High fluid intake negates the positive effects of diuretics and induces hyponatraemia.

Community and social support

- Community support is particularly important for elderly or functionally restricted patients with chronic heart failure
- Support may help to improve the quality of life and reduce admission rates
- Social services support and community based interventions, with advice and assistance for close relatives, are also important

---

Managing cachexia in chronic heart failure

Combined management by physician and dietician is recommended
- Alter size and frequency of meals
- Ensure a higher energy diet
- Supplement diet with (a) water soluble vitamins (loss associated with diuresis), (b) fat soluble vitamins (levels reduced as a result of poor absorption), and (c) fish oils

---

Date								
Pulse								
BP (lying)								
BP (standing)								
Urine								
Weight								
Drug 1								
Drug 2								
Drug 3								
Drug 4								
Drug 5								
Drug 6								
Serum urea/creatinine								
Serum potassium								
Other investigations								
Next visit								
Doctor's signature								

Heart failure cooperation card: patients and doctors are able to monitor changes in clinical signs (including weight), drug treatment, and baseline investigations. Patients should be encouraged to monitor their weight between clinic visits

---

Commonly consumed processed foods that have a high sodium content

- Cheese
- Sausages
- Crisps, salted peanuts
- Milk and white chocolate
- Tinned soup and tinned vegetables
- Ham, bacon, tinned meat (eg corned beef)
- Tinned fish (eg sardines, salmon, tuna)
- Smoked fish

Fresh produce, such as fruit, vegetables, eggs, and fish, has a relatively low salt content

Exercise training and rehabilitation

Exercise training has been shown to benefit patients with heart failure: patients show an improvement in symptoms, a greater sense of wellbeing, and better functional capacity. Exercise does not, however, result in obvious improvement in cardiac function.

All stable patients with heart failure should be encouraged to participate in a supervised, simple exercise programme. Although bed rest ("armchair treatment") may be appropriate in patients with acute heart failure, regular exercise should be encouraged in patients with chronic heart failure. Indeed, chronic immobility may result in loss of muscle mass in the lower limb and generalised physical deconditioning, leading to a further reduction in exercise capacity and a predisposition to thromboembolism. Deconditioning itself may be detrimental, with peripheral alterations and central abnormalities leading to vasoconstriction, further deterioration in left ventricular function, and greater reduction in functional capacity.

Importantly, regular exercise has the potential to slow or stop this process and exert beneficial effects on the autonomic profile, with reduced sympathetic activity and enhanced vagal tone, thus reversing some of the adverse consequences of heart failure. Large prospective clinical trials will establish whether these beneficial effects improve prognosis and reduce the incidence of sudden death in patients with chronic heart failure.

Regular exercise should therefore be advocated in stable patients as there is the potential for improvements in exercise tolerance and quality of life, without deleterious effects on left ventricular function. Cardiac rehabilitation services offer benefit to this group, and patients should be encouraged to develop their own regular exercise routine, including walking, cycling, and swimming. Nevertheless, patients should know their limits, and excessive fatigue or breathlessness should be avoided. In the first instance, a structured walking programme would be the easiest to adopt.

Beneficial effects of exercise in chronic heart failure

Has positive effects on:
- Skeletal muscle
- Autonomic function
- Endothelial function
- Neurohormonal function
- Insulin sensitivity

No positive effects on survival have been shown

Effects of deconditioning in heart failure

Peripheral alterations	Increased peripheral vascular resistance; impaired oxygen utilisation during exercise
Abnormalities of autonomic control	Enhanced sympathetic activation; vagal withdrawal; reduced baroreflex sensitivity
Skeletal muscle abnormalities	Reduced mass and composition
Reduced functional capacity	Reduced exercise tolerance; reduced peak oxygen consumption
Psychological effects	Reduced activity; reduced overall sense of wellbeing

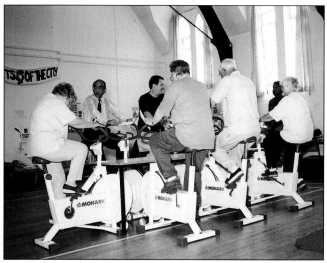

Exercise class for group of patients with heart failure (published with permission of participants)

Treatment of underlying disease

Treatment should also be aimed at slowing or reversing any underlying disease process.

Hypertension

Good blood pressure control is essential, and angiotensin converting enzyme inhibitors are the drugs of choice in patients with impaired systolic function, in view of their beneficial effects on slowing disease progression and improving prognosis. In cases of isolated diastolic dysfunction, either β blockers or calcium channel blockers with rate limiting properties—for example, verapamil, diltiazem—have theoretical advantages. If severe left ventricular hypertrophy is the cause of diastolic dysfunction, however, an angiotensin converting enzyme inhibitor may be more effective at inducing regression of left ventricular hypertrophy. Angiotensin II receptor antagonists should be considered as an alternative if cough that is induced by angiotensin converting enzyme inhibitors is problematic.

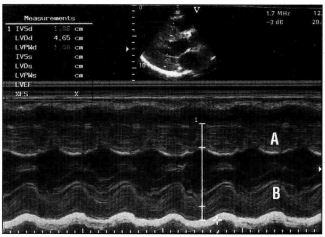

M mode echocardiogram showing left ventricular hypertrophy in hypertensive patient (A=interventricular septum; B=posterior wall of left ventricle)

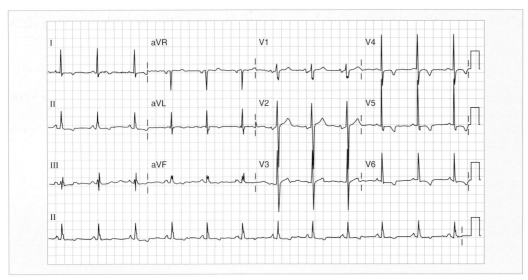

Electrocardiogram showing left ventricular hypertrophy on voltage criteria, with associated T wave and ST changes in the lateral leads ("strain pattern")

Surgery

If coronary heart disease is the underlying cause of chronic heart failure and if cardiac ischaemia is present, the patient may benefit from coronary revascularisation, including coronary angioplasty or coronary artery bypass grafting. Revascularisation may also improve the function of previously hibernating myocardium. Valve replacement or valve repair should be considered in patients with haemodynamically important primary valve disease.

Cardiac transplantation is now established as the treatment of choice for some patients with severe heart failure who remain symptomatic despite intensive medical treatment. It is associated with a one year survival of about 90% and a 10 year survival of 50-60%, although it is limited by the availability of donor organs. Transplantation should be considered in younger patients (aged <60 years) who are without severe concomitant disease (for example, renal failure or malignancy).

Bradycardias are managed with conventional permanent cardiac pacing, although a role is emerging for biventricular cardiac pacing in some patients with resistant severe congestive heart failure. Implantable cardiodefibrillators are well established in the treatment of some patients with resistant life threatening ventricular arrhythmias. New surgical approaches such as cardiomyoplasty and ventricular reduction surgery (Batista procedure) are rarely used owing to the high associated morbidity and mortality and the lack of conclusive trial evidence of substantial benefit.

The box about managing cachexia is based on recommendations from the Scottish Intercollegiate Guidelines Network (SIGN) (publication No 35, 1999).

Role of surgery in heart failure

Type of surgery	Reason
Coronary revascularisation (PTCA, CABG)	Angina, reversible ischaemia, hibernating myocardium
Valve replacement (or repair)	Significant valve disease (aortic stenosis, mitral regurgitation)
Permanent pacemakers and implantable cardiodefibrillators	Bradycardias; resistant ventricular arrhythmias
Cardiac transplantation	End stage heart failure
Ventricular assist devices	Short term ventricular support—eg awaiting transplantation
Novel surgical techniques	Limited role (high mortality, limited evidence of substantial benefit)

PTCA = percutaneous transluminal coronary angioplasty; CABG = coronary artery bypass graft.

Key references

- Demakis JG, Proskey A, Rahimtoola SH, Jamil M, Sutton GC, Rosen KM, et al. The natural course of alcoholic cardiomyopathy. *Ann Intern Med* 1974;80:293-7.
- The Task Force of the Working Group on Heart Failure of the European Society of Cardiology. Guidelines on the treatment of heart failure. *Eur Heart J* 1997;18:736-53.
- Kostis JB, Rosen RC, Cosgrove NM, Shindler DM, Wilson AC. Nonpharmacologic therapy improves functional and emotional status in congestive heart failure. *Chest* 1994;106:996-1001.
- McKelvie RS, Teo KK, McCartney N, Humen D, Montague T, Yusuf S. Effects of exercise training in patients with congestive heart failure: a critical review. *J Am Coll Cardiol* 1995;25:789-96.

7   Management: diuretics, ACE inhibitors, and nitrates

M K Davies, C R Gibbs, G Y H Lip

In the past 15 years several large scale, randomised controlled trials have revolutionised the management of patients with chronic heart failure. Although it is clear that some drugs improve symptoms, others offer both symptomatic and prognostic benefits, and the management of heart failure should be aimed at improving both quality of life and survival.

Diuretics and angiotensin converting enzyme (ACE) inhibitors, when combined with non-pharmacological measures, remain the basis of treatment in patients with congestive heart failure. Digoxin has a possible role in some of these patients, however, and the potential benefits of β blockers and spironolactone (an aldosterone antagonist) in chronic heart failure are now increasingly recognised.

Diuretics

Diuretics are effective in providing symptomatic relief and remain the first line treatment, particularly in the presence of oedema. Nevertheless, there is no direct evidence that loop and thiazide diuretics confer prognostic benefit in patients with congestive heart failure.

Loop diuretics

Loop diuretics—frusemide (furosemide) and bumetanide—have a powerful diuretic action, increasing the excretion of sodium and water via their action on the ascending limb of the loop of Henle. They have a rapid onset of action (intravenously 5 minutes, orally 1-2 hours; duration of action 4-6 hours). Oral absorption of frusemide may be reduced in congestive heart failure, although the pharmacokinetics of bumetanide may allow improved bioavailability.

Patients receiving high dose diuretics (frusemide ≥80 mg or equivalent) should be monitored for renal and electrolyte abnormalities. Hypokalaemia, which may precipitate arrhythmias, should be avoided, and potassium supplementation, or concomitant treatment with a potassium sparing agent, should generally be used unless contraindicated—for example, in renal dysfunction with potassium retention. Acute gout is a relatively common adverse effect of treatment with high dose intravenous diuretics.

Thiazide diuretics

Thiazides—such as bendrofluazide (bendroflumethiazide)—act on the cortical diluting segment of the nephron. They are often ineffective in elderly people, owing to the age related and heart failure mediated reduction in glomerular filtration rate. Hyponatraemia and hypokalaemia are commonly associated with higher doses of thiazide diuretics, and potassium supplementation, or concomitant treatment with a potassium sparing agent, is usually needed with high dose thiazide therapy.

In some patients with chronic severe congestive heart failure, particularly in the presence of chronic renal impairment, oedema may persist despite conventional oral doses (frusemide 40-160 mg daily) of loop diuretics. In these patients, a thiazide diuretic (for example, bendrofluazide) or a thiazide-like diuretic (for example, metolazone) may be combined with a loop diuretic. This combination blocks reabsorption of sodium at different sites in the nephron

---

Aims of heart failure management

To achieve improvement in symptoms
- Diuretics
- Digoxin
- ACE inhibitors

To achieve improvement in survival
- ACE inhibitors
- β blockers (for example, carvedilol and bisoprolol)
- Oral nitrates plus hydralazine
- Spironolactone

In general, diuretics should be introduced at a low dose and the dose increased according to the clinical response. There are dangers, however, in either undertreating or overtreating patients with diuretics, and regular review is necessary

---

How to use diuretics in advanced heart failure

- Optimise diuretic dose
- Consider combination diuretic treatment with a loop and thiazide (or thiazide-like) diuretic
- Consider combining a low dose of spironolactone with an ACE inhibitor, provided that there is no evidence of hyperkalaemia
- Administer loop diuretics (either as a bolus or a continuous infusion) intravenously

---

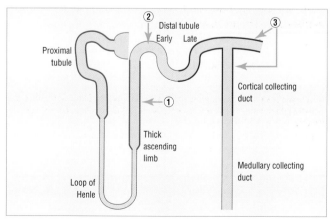

Diagram of nephron showing sites of action of different diuretic classes: 1=loop (eg frusemide); 2=thiazide (eg bendrofluazide); and 3=potassium sparing (eg amiloride)

("double nephron blockade"), and this synergistic action leads to a greater diuretic effect. The incidence of associated metabolic abnormalities is, however, increased, and such treatment should be started only under close supervision. In some patients, a large diuretic effect may occur soon after a combination regimen (loop diuretic plus either thiazide or metalozone) has been started. It is advisable, therefore, to consider such a combination treatment on a twice weekly basis, at least initially.

Potassium sparing diuretics

Amiloride acts on the distal nephron, while spironolactone is a competitive aldosterone inhibitor. Potassium sparing diuretics have generally been avoided in patients receiving ACE inhibitors, owing to the potential risk of hyperkalaemia. Nevertheless, a recent randomised placebo controlled study, the randomised aldactone evaluation study (RALES), reported that hyperkalaemia is uncommon when low dose spironolactone (≤25 mg daily) is combined with an ACE inhibitor. Risk factors for developing hyperkalaemia include spironolactone dose >50 mg/day, high doses of ACE inhibitor, or evidence of renal impairment. It is recommended that measurement of the serum creatinine and potassium concentrations is performed within 5-7 days of the addition of a potassium sparing diuretic to an ACE inhibitor until the levels are stable, and then every one to three months.

ACE inhibitors

ACE inhibitors have consistently shown beneficial effects on mortality, morbidity, and quality of life in large scale, prospective clinical trials and are indicated in all stages of symptomatic heart failure resulting from impaired left ventricular systolic function.

Mechanisms of action

ACE inhibitors inhibit the production of angiotensin II, a potent vasoconstrictor and growth promoter, and increase concentrations of the vasodilator bradykinin by inhibiting its degradation. Bradykinin has been shown to have beneficial effects associated with the release of nitric oxide and prostacyclin, which may contribute to the positive haemodynamic effects of the ACE inhibitors. Bradykinin may also be responsible, however, for some of the adverse effects, such as dry cough, hypotension, and angio-oedema.

ACE inhibitors also reduce the activity of the sympathetic nervous system as angiotensin II promotes the release of noradrenaline and inhibits its reuptake. In addition, they also improve β receptor density (causing their up regulation), variation in heart rate, baroreceptor function, and autonomic function (including vagal tone).

Clinical effects

Symptomatic left ventricular dysfunction
ACE inhibitors, when added to diuretics, improve symptoms, exercise tolerance, and survival and reduce hospital admission rates in chronic heart failure.

These beneficial effects are apparent in all grades of systolic heart failure—that is, mild to moderate chronic heart failure (as evident, for example, in the Munich mild heart failure study, the vasodilator heart failure trials (V-HeFT), and the studies of left ventricular dysfunction treatment trial (SOLVD-T)) and severe chronic heart failure (as, for example, in the first cooperative north Scandinavian enalapril survival study (CONSENSUS I).

The two main potassium sparing diuretics, amiloride and spironolactone, have a weak diuretic action when used alone; amiloride is most commonly used in fixed dose combinations with a loop diuretic—for example, co-amilofruse

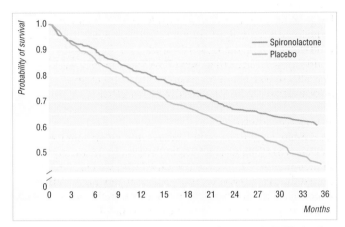

Survival curve for randomised aldactone evaluation study (RALES) showing 30% reduction in all cause mortality when spironolactone (up to 25 mg) was added to conventional treatment in patients with severe (New York Heart Association class IV) chronic heart failure

Guidelines for using ACE inhibitors

- Stop potassium supplements and potassium sparing diuretics
- Omit (or reduce) diuretics for 24 hours before first dose
- Advise patient to sit or lie down for 2-4 hours after first dose
- Start low doses (for example, captopril 6.25 mg twice daily, enalapril 2.5 mg once daily, lisinopril 2.5 mg once daily)
- Review after 1-2 weeks to reassess symptoms, blood pressure, and renal chemistry and electrolytes
- Increase dose unless there has been a rise in serum creatinine concentration (to >200 μmol/l) or potassium concentration (to >5.0 mmol/l)
- Titrate to maximum tolerated dose, reassessing blood pressure and renal chemistry and electrolytes after each dose titration

If patient is "high risk" consider hospital admission to start treatment

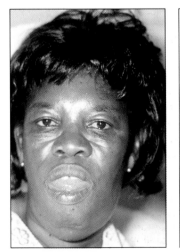
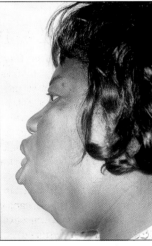

Front view and side view of woman with angio-oedema related to treatment with ACE inhibitors (published with permission of patient)

Asymptomatic left ventricular dysfunction

ACE inhibitors have also been shown to be effective in asymptomatic patients with left ventricular systolic dysfunction. The studies of left ventricular dysfunction prevention trial (SOLVD-P) confirmed the benefit of ACE inhibitors in asymptomatic left ventricular systolic dysfunction, where enalapril reduced the development of heart failure and related hospital admissions.

Left ventricular dysfunction after myocardial infarction

Large scale, randomised controlled trials—for example, the acute infarction ramipril efficacy (AIRE) study, the survival and ventricular enlargement (SAVE) study, and the trial of trandolapril cardiac evaluation (TRACE)—have shown lower mortality in patients with impaired systolic function after myocardial infarction, irrespective of symptoms.

Slowing disease progression

ACE inhibitors also seem to influence the natural course of chronic heart failure. The Munich mild heart failure study showed that ACE inhibitors combined with standard treatment slowed the progression of heart failure in patients with mild symptoms, with significantly fewer patients in the active treatment group developing severe heart failure.

Doses and tolerability

ACE inhibitors should be started at a low dose and gradually titrated to the highest tolerated maintenance level. The recent prospective assessment trial of lisinopril and survival (ATLAS) randomised patients with symptomatic heart failure to low dose (2.5-5 mg daily) or high dose (32.5-35 mg daily) lisinopril, and, although there was no significant mortality difference, high dose treatment was associated with a significant reduction in the combined end point of all cause mortality and all cause admissions to hospital. Adverse effects of the ACE inhibitors include cough, dizziness, and a deterioration in renal function, although the overall incidence of hypotension and renal impairment in the CONSENSUS and SOLVD studies was only 5%. Angio-oedema related to ACE inhibitors is rare, although more common in patients of Afro-Caribbean origin than in other ethnic groups.

ACE inhibitors can therefore be regarded as the cornerstone of treatment in patients with all grades of symptomatic heart failure and in patients with asymptomatic left ventricular dysfunction. Every attempt should be made to provide this treatment for patients, unless it is contraindicated, and to use adequate doses.

Angiotensin receptor antagonists

Orally active angiotensin II type 1 receptor antagonists, such as losartan, represent a new class of agents that offer an alternative method of blocking the renin-angiotensin system. The effects of angiotensin II receptor antagonists on haemodynamics, neuroendocrine activity, and exercise tolerance resemble those of ACE inhibitors, although it still remains to be established fully whether these receptor antagonists are an effective substitute for ACE inhibitors in patients with chronic heart failure.

The evaluation of losartan in the elderly (ELITE) study compared losartan with captopril in patients aged 65 or over with mild to severe congestive heart failure. Although the ELITE study was designed as a tolerability study, and survival was not the primary end point, it did report a reduction in all cause mortality (4.8% *v* 8.7%) in patients treated with losartan.

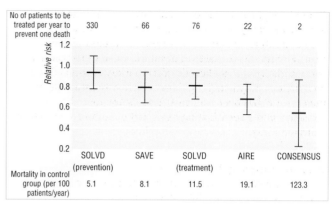

ACE inhibitors in left ventricular dysfunction: best benefit for ACE inhibitors in higher risk group

---

Meta-analysis of effects of ACE inhibitors on mortality and admissions in chronic heart failure

No of trials	Total No of patients	Placebo (%)	Active treatment (%)	Risk reduction (%)	P value
32	7105	32.6	22.4	35	<0.001

ACE inhibitors: high risk patients warranting hospital admission for start of treatment

- Severe heart failure (NYHA class IV) or decompensated heart failure
- Low systolic blood pressure (<100 mm Hg)
- Resting tachycardia >100 beats/minute
- Low serum sodium concentration (<130 mmol/l)
- Other vasodilator treatment
- Severe chronic obstructive airways disease and pulmonary heart disease (cor pulmonale)

Doses of ACE inhibitors used in large controlled trials

Trial	ACE inhibitor	Target dose (mg)	Mean daily dose (mg)
CONSENSUS	Enalapril	20*	18.4
V-HeFT II	Enalapril	10*	15.0
SOLVD	Enalapril	10*	16.6
SAVE	Captopril	50†	NA

*Twice daily; †three times daily. NA=information not available.

Recommended maintenance doses of ACE inhibitors

Drug	Starting dose (mg)	Maintenance dose (mg)
Captopril	6.25†	25-50†
Enalapril	2.5‡	10*
Lisinopril	2.5‡	5-20‡
Quinapril	2.5-5‡	5-10*
Perindopril	2‡	4‡
Ramipril	1.25-2.5‡	2.5-5*
Trandolapril	0.5‡	2-4‡

*Twice daily; †three times daily; ‡once daily.

Important limitations of the ELITE study included the limited size and the relatively short follow up. However, the recently reported ELITE II mortality study failed to show that treatment with losartan was superior to captopril, although it confirmed improved tolerability with losartan.

ACE inhibitors, therefore, remain the treatment of choice in patients with left ventricular systolic dysfunction, although angiotensin II receptor antagonists are an appropriate alternative in patients who develop intolerable side effects from ACE inhibitors.

Oral nitrates and hydralazine

The V-HeFT trials showed a survival benefit from combined treatment with nitrates and hydralazine in patients with symptomatic heart failure (New York Heart Association class II-III). The V-HeFT II trial also showed a modest improvement in exercise capacity, although the nitrate and hydralazine combination was less well tolerated than enalapril, owing to the dose related adverse effects (dizziness and headaches). There is no reproducible evidence of symptomatic improvement from other randomised placebo controlled trials, however, and survival rates were higher with ACE inhibitors than with the nitrate and hydralazine combination (V-HeFT II trial).

In general, oral nitrates should be considered in patients with angina and impaired left ventricular systolic function. The combination of nitrates and hydralazine is an alternative regimen in patients with severe renal impairment, in whom ACE inhibitors and angiotensin II receptor antagonists are contraindicated. Although it is rational to consider the addition of a combination of nitrates and hydralazine in patients who continue to have severe symptoms despite optimal doses of ACE inhibitors, no large scale trials have shown an additive effect of these combinations.

Other vasodilators

Long acting dihydropyridine calcium channel blockers generally have neutral effects in heart failure, although others, such as diltiazem and verapamil, have negatively inotropic and chronotropic properties, with the potential to exacerbate heart failure. Two recent trials of the newer calcium channel blockers amlodipine (the prospective randomised amlodipine survival evaluation (PRAISE) trial) and felodipine (V-HeFT III) in patients with heart failure suggest that long acting calcium antagonists may have beneficial effects in non-ischaemic dilated cardiomyopathy, although further studies are in progress—for example, PRAISE II. Importantly, these studies indicate that amlodipine and felodipine seem to be safe in patients with congestive heart failure and could therefore be used to treat angina and hypertension in this group of patients.

The two tables on recommended doses of ACE inhibitors are adapted and reproduced with permission from Remme WJ (*Eur Heart J* 1997;18: 736-53). The meta-analysis table is adapted and used with permission from Garg R et al (*JAMA* 1995;273:1450-6). The graph showing the benefit of ACE inhibitors in left ventricular dysfunction is adapted from Davey Smith et al (*BMJ* 1994;308:73-4).

ELITE II study: the losartan heart failure survival study

- Multicentre, randomised, parallel group trial of captopril *v* losartan in chronic stable heart failure
- 3152 patients; age >60 years (mean age 71.5 years); NYHA class II-IV heart failure; mean follow up of 2 years
- No significant difference in all cause mortality between the captopril group (15.9%) and losartan group (17.7%)
- Better tolerability with losartan (withdrawal rate 9.4%) than with captopril (14.5%)

Vasodilator heart failure (V-HeFT) studies

Study	Comparison	NYHA class*	Outcome
V-HeFT I	Hydralazine plus isosorbide dinitrate *v* placebo	II, III	Improved mortality with active treatment
V-HeFT II	Hydralazine plus isosorbide dinitrate *v* enalapril	II, III	Enalapril superior to hydralazine plus isosorbide dinitrate for survival

*I = asymptomatic, II = mild, III = moderate, IV = severe.

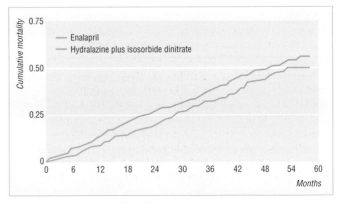

Cumulative mortality in V-HeFT II trial: enalapril *v* hydralazine plus isosorbide dinitrate in patients with congestive heart failure (mild to moderate)

Key references

- Cohn JN, Johnson G, Ziesche S, Cobb F, Francis G, Tristani F, et al. A comparison of enalapril with hydralazine-isosorbide dinitrate in the treatment of chronic congestive heart failure. *N Engl J Med* 1991;325:303-10.
- Cohn JN, Ziesche S, Smith R, Anand I, Dunkman WB, Loeb H, et al. Effect of the calcium antagonist felodipine as supplementary vasodilator therapy in patients with chronic heart failure treated with enalapril. V-HeFT III. *Circulation* 1997;96:856-63.
- Packer M, O'Connor CM, Ghali JK, Pressler ML, Carson PE, Belkin RN, et al. Effect of amlodipine on morbidity and mortality in severe chronic heart failure. *N Engl J Med* 1996;335:1107-14.
- Pitt B, Segal R, Martinez FA, Meurers G, Cowley AJ, Thomas I, et al. Randomised trial of losartan versus captopril in patients over 65 with heart failure. *Lancet* 1997;349:747-52.
- Remme WJ. The treatment of heart failure. The Task Force of the Working Group on Heart Failure of the European Society of Cardiology. *Eur Heart J* 1997;18:736-53.
- Pitt B, Zannad F, Remme WJ, Cody R, Castaigne A, Perez A, et al. The effect of spironolactone on morbidity and mortality in patients with severe heart failure. *N Engl J Med* 1999;341:709-17.

8   Management: digoxin and other inotropes, β blockers, and antiarrhythmic and antithrombotic treatment

C R Gibbs, M K Davies, G Y H Lip

Digoxin

Use of digoxin for heart failure varies between countries across Europe, with high rates in Germany and low rates in the United Kingdom. It is potentially invaluable in patients with atrial fibrillation and coexistent heart failure, improving control of the ventricular rate and allowing more effective filling of the ventricle. Digoxin is also used in patients with chronic heart failure secondary to left ventricular systolic impairment, in sinus rhythm, who remain symptomatic despite optimal doses of diuretics and angiotensin converting enzyme inhibitors, where it acts as an inotrope.

Evidence of symptomatic benefit from digoxin in patients with chronic heart failure in sinus rhythm has been reported in several randomised placebo controlled trials and several smaller trials. The RADIANCE and PROVED trials, for example, reported that the withdrawal of digoxin from patients with congestive heart failure who had already been treated with the drug was associated with worsening heart failure and increased hospital readmission rates. The Digitalis Investigation Group's large study found that digoxin was associated with a symptomatic improvement in patients with congestive heart failure, when added to treatment with diuretics and angiotensin converting enzyme inhibitors. Importantly, there were greater absolute and relative benefits in the patients who had resistant symptoms and more severe impairment of left ventricular systolic function. However, although there was a reduction in the combined end points of admission and mortality resulting from heart failure, there was no significant improvement in overall survival. β Blockers were used rarely in the Digitalis Investigation Group's study, and as a result it is not clear whether digoxin is additive to both the β blockers and angiotensin converting enzyme inhibitors in congestive heart failure.

Digoxin should be considered in patients with sinus rhythm plus *(a)* continued symptoms of heart failure despite optimal doses of diuretics and angiotensin converting enzyme inhibitors; *(b)* severe left ventricular systolic dysfunction with cardiac dilatation; or *(c)* recurrent hospital admissions for heart failure

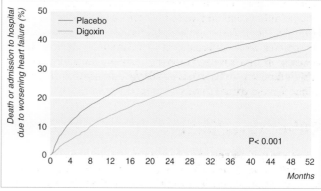

Incidence of death or admission to hospital due to worsening heart failure in two groups of patients: those receiving digoxin and those receiving placebo (Digitalis Investigation Group's study—see key references box at end of article)

Digoxin: practical aspects

- Ensure a maintenance dose of 125-375 µg (0.125-0.375 mg) daily
- Give a reduced maintenance dose in elderly people, when renal impairment is present, and when used with drugs that increase digoxin concentrations (amiodarone, verapamil)
- Concentrations should be monitored especially in cases of uncertainty about whether therapeutic levels have been achieved (range 6 hours after dose: 1.2-1.9 ng/ml)
- Monitor potassium concentrations (avoid hypokalaemia) and renal function
- Digoxin toxicity may be associated with: *(a)* adverse symptoms (for example, nausea, vomiting, headache, confusion, visual symptoms); and *(b)* arrhythmias (for example, atrioventricular junctional rhythms, atrial tachycardia, atrioventricular block, ventricular tachycardia)
- Serious toxicity should be treated by correcting potassium concentrations and with drugs such as β blockers and glycoside binding agents (cholestyramine), and in severe cases specific digoxin antibodies (Digibind)

Source of information: Uretsky et al (*J Am Coll Cardiol* 1993;22:955) and Packer et al (*N Engl J Med* 1993;329:1)

Study of effect of digoxin on mortality and morbidity in patients with heart failure*

Number of participants: 6800

Design: prospective, randomised, double blind, placebo controlled

Participants: left ventricular ejection fraction <45%

Intervention: randomised to digoxin (0.125-0.500 mg) or placebo; follow up at 37 months

Results:
- Reduced admissions to hospital owing to heart failure (greater absolute and relative benefits in the patients with resistant symptoms and more severe impairment of left ventricular systolic function)
- No effect on overall survival

*The Digitalis Investigation Group's study (see key references box)

Other inotropes

The potential role of inotropic agents other than digoxin in chronic heart failure has been addressed in several studies. Although these drugs seem to improve symptoms in some patients, most have been associated with an increase in mortality.

For example, the PRIME II trial (a prospective randomised study) examined ibopamine, a weak inotrope, in patients with chronic heart failure who were already receiving standard treatment. An excess mortality was shown, however, particularly in those with severe symptoms; this was possibly related to an excess of arrhythmias. In addition, a previous trial evaluating intermittent dobutamine infusions in patients with chronic heart failure was stopped prematurely because of excess mortality in the group taking dobutamine. Xamoterol, a β receptor antagonist with mild agonist inotropic effects, also failed to show any positive benefits in patients with heart failure.

In overall terms, no evidence exists at present to support the use of oral catecholamine receptor (or postreceptor pathway) stimulants in the treatment of chronic heart failure. Digoxin remains the only (albeit weak) positive inotrope that is valuable in the management of chronic heart failure.

β Blockers

β Adrenoceptor blockers have traditionally been avoided in patients with heart failure due to their negative inotropic effects. However, there is now considerable clinical evidence to support the use of β blockers in patients with chronic stable heart failure resulting from left ventricular systolic dysfunction. Recent randomised controlled trials in patients with chronic heart failure have reported that combining β blockers with conventional treatment with diuretics and angiotensin converting enzyme inhibitors results in improvements in left ventricular function, symptoms, and survival, as well as a reduction in admissions to hospital.

Recently, two randomised controlled trials have studied the effects of carvedilol, a β blocker with α blocking and vasodilator properties, in patients with symptomatic heart failure. The US multicentre carvedilol study programme was stopped early because of a highly significant (65%) mortality benefit in patients receiving carvedilol, when compared to placebo, and the Australia/New Zealand heart failure study reported a 41% reduction in the combined primary end point of all cause hospital admission and mortality. Bisoprolol has also been studied, and, although the first cardiac insufficiency bisoprolol study (CIBIS I) reported a trend towards a reduction in mortality and need for cardiac transplantation, there was no conclusive survival benefit. The recent CIBIS II study, however, was stopped prematurely because of the beneficial effects of active treatment on both morbidity and mortality. Metoprolol has also shown similar prognostic advantages in the metoprolol randomised intervention trial in heart failure (MERIT-HF), which was also stopped early. In summary, evidence is now

Meta-analysis of effects of β blockers on mortality and admissions to hospital in chronic heart failure

No of trials (total No of patients)	% receiving placebo	% receiving active treatment	Risk reduction (%)	P value
18 (3023)	24.6	15.8	38	<0.001

Inotropic drugs associated with increased mortality in chronic heart failure

Drug	Class	Inotropic activity
Xamoterol	β Receptor antagonist	Mild
Dobutamine	Dopamine, α, and β receptor antagonist	Strong
Ibopamine	Dopamine, α, and β receptor antagonist	Weak
Amrinone	Phosphodiesterase inhibitor	Strong
Enoximone	Phosphodiesterase inhibitor	Strong
Flosequinan	Attenuates inositol triphosphate	Weak
Milrinone	Phosphodiesterase inhibitor	Strong
Vesnarinone	Phosphodiesterase inhibitor	Mild

Potential mechanisms and benefits of β blockers: improved left ventricular function; reduced sympathetic tone; improved autonomic nervous system balance; up regulation of β adrenergic receptors; reduction in arrhythmias, ischaemia, further infarction, myocardial fibrosis, and apoptosis

Randomised, placebo controlled β blocker trials in congestive heart failure

Study	Treatment	NYHA class*	Outcome
MDC	Metoprolol	II, III	Improved clinical state without effect on survival. Reduction in need for transplantation in patients with dilated cardiomyopathy
CIBIS I	Bisoprolol	II, III	Trend (non-significant) towards improved survival
ANZ trial	Carvedilol	I, II	Carvedilol superior to placebo for morbidity and mortality
Carvedilol (US)	Carvedilol	II, III	Carvedilol superior to placebo for morbidity and mortality
CIBIS II	Bisoprolol	III, IV	Bisoprolol superior to placebo for morbidity and mortality
MERIT-HF	Metoprolol	II, III	Metoprolol superior to placebo for morbidity and mortality

Placebo groups in all trials received appropriate conventional treatment (diuretics alone; diuretics plus either digoxin or angiotensin converting enzyme inhibitors; or diuretics plus digoxin and angiotensin converting enzyme inhibitors). Trials still in progress: COMET (carvedilol v metoprolol) and COPERNICUS (carvedilol in severe chronic heart failure).
*Classification of the New York Heart Association (I = no symptoms, II = mild, III = moderate, IV = severe).

available to support the use of β blockers in chronic heart failure, as the benefits supplement those already obtained from angiotensin converting enzyme inhibitors.

Carvedilol is now licensed in the United Kingdom for use in mild to moderate chronic stable heart failure, although at present its use is still not recommended in patients with severe symptoms (New York Heart Association class IV). This latter group has been underrepresented in the trials to date.

In general, β blockers should be started at very low doses, with the dose being slowly increased, under expert supervision, to the target dose if tolerated. In the short term there may be a deterioration in symptoms, which may improve with alterations in other treatment, particularly diuretics.

Summary of the cardiac insufficiency bisoprolol study II (CIBIS II)*

- Randomised, double blind, parallel group study
- 2647 participants (class III-IV (moderate to severe) according to classification of the New York Heart Association)
- Bisoprolol, increased in dose to a maximum of 10 mg a day
- Trial stopped because of significant mortality benefit in patients treated with bisoprolol:

(*a*) 32% reduction in all cause mortality

(*b*) 32% reduction in admissions to hospital for worsening heart failure

(*c*) 42% reduction in sudden death

*CIBIS II Investigators and Committee (*Lancet* 1999;353:9-13)

Dose and titration of β blockers in large, placebo controlled heart failure trials

β Blocker	Initial dose (mg)	Weekly titration schedule: total daily dose (mg)									Target total daily dose (mg)
		1	2	3	4	5	6	7	8–11	12–15	
Metoprolol (MDC trial)	5	10	15	20	50	75	100	150	NI	NI	100–150
Carvedilol (US trials)	3.125	6.25	NI	12.5	NI	25	NI	50	NI	NI	50
Bisoprolol (CIBIS II)	1.25	1.25	2.5	3.75	5	5	5	5	7.5	10	10

References: Waagstein F et al (*Lancet* 1993;342:1442-6), Packer M et al (*N Engl J Med* 1996;334:1349-55), and CIBIS II Investigators and Committee (*Lancet* 1999;353:9-13).
NI = no increase in dose.

Antithrombotic treatment

In patients with chronic heart failure the incidence of stroke and thromboembolism is significantly higher in the presence of atrial and left ventricular dilatation, particularly in severe left ventricular dysfunction. Nevertheless, there is conflicting evidence of benefit from routine treatment of patients with heart failure who are in sinus rhythm with antithrombotic treatment, although anticoagulation should be considered in the presence of mobile ventricular thrombus, atrial fibrillation, and severe cardiac impairment. Large scale, prospective randomised controlled trials of antithrombotic treatment in heart failure are in progress, such as the WATCH study (a trial of warfarin and antiplatelet therapy); the full results are awaited with interest.

The combination of atrial fibrillation and heart failure (or evidence of left ventricular systolic dysfunction on echocardiography) is associated with a particularly high risk of thromboembolism, which is reduced by long term treatment with warfarin. Aspirin seems to have little effect on the risk of thromboembolism and overall mortality in such patients.

Echocardiogram showing thrombus at left ventricular apex in patient with dilated cardiomyopathy (A=thrombus, B=left ventricle, C=left atrium)

Antiarrhythmic treatment

Chronic heart failure and atrial fibrillation

Restoration and long term maintenance of sinus rhythm is less successful in the presence of severe structural heart disease, particularly when the atrial fibrillation is longstanding. In patients with a deterioration in symptoms that is associated with recent onset atrial fibrillation, treatment with amiodarone increases the long term success rate of cardioversion. Digoxin is otherwise appropriate for controlling ventricular rate in most patients with heart failure and chronic atrial fibrillation, with the addition of amiodarone in resistant cases.

The use of class I antiarrhythmic agents in patients with atrial fibrillation and chronic heart failure substantially increases the risk of mortality

Chronic heart failure and ventricular arrhythmias

Ventricular arrhythmias are a common cause of death in severe heart failure. Precipitating or aggravating factors should thus be addressed, including electrolyte disturbance (for example, hypokalaemia, hypomagnesaemia), digoxin toxicity, drugs causing electrical instability (for example, antiarrhythmic drugs, antidepressants), and continued or recurrent myocardial ischaemia.

Amiodarone is effective for the symptomatic control of ventricular arrhythmias in chronic heart failure, although most studies have reported that long term antiarrhythmic treatment with amiodarone has a neutral effect on survival. An Argentinian trial (the GESICA study) of empirical amiodarone in patients with chronic heart failure reported, however, that active treatment was associated with a 28% reduction in total mortality, although this trial included a high incidence of patients with non-ischaemic heart failure. In contrast, in the survival trial of antiarrhythmic therapy in congestive heart failure (CHF-STAT), amiodarone did not improve overall survival, although there was a significant (46%) reduction in cardiac death and admission to hospital in the patients with non-ischaemic chronic heart failure.

In general, amiodarone should probably be reserved for patients with chronic heart failure who also have symptomatic ventricular arrhythmias. Interest has also developed in implantable cardioverter defibrillators, which reduce the risk of sudden death in high risk patients with ventricular arrhythmias (MADIT and AVID studies), although the role of these devices in patients with chronic heart failure still remains to be established.

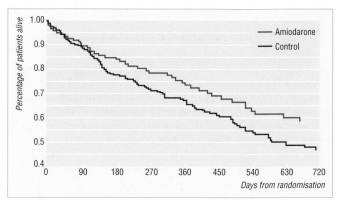

Survival curves from GESICA trial (see key references box), showing difference between patients taking amiodarone and controls

Key references

- Australia/New Zealand Heart Failure Research Collaborative Group. Randomized, placebo-controlled trial of carvedilol in patients with congestive heart failure due to ischaemic heart disease. *Lancet* 1997;349:375-80.
- Lip GYH. Intracardiac thrombus formation in cardiac impairment: investigation and the role of anticoagulant therapy. *Postgrad Med J* 1996;72:731-8.
- Massie BM, Fisher SG, Radford M, Deedwania PC, Singh BN, Fletcher RD, et al for the CHF-STAT Investigators. Effect of amiodarone on clinical status and left ventricular function in patients with congestive heart failure. *Circulation* 1996;93:2128-34.
- MERIT-HF Study Group. Effect of metoprolol CR/XL in chronic heart failure: metoprolol CR/XL randomised intervention trial in congestive heart failure (MERIT-HF). *Lancet* 1999;353:2001-7.
- Doval HC, Nul DR, Grancelli HO, Perrone SV, Bortman GR, Curiel R, et al. Randomised trial of low-dose amiodarone in severe congestive heart failure [GESICA trial]. *Lancet* 1994;344:493-8.
- Packer M, Bristow MR, Cohn JN, Colucci WS, Fowler MB, Gilbert EM, et al. Effect of carvedilol on morbidity and mortality in patients with chronic heart failure. *N Engl J Med* 1996;334:1349-55.
- Digitalis Investigation Group. The effect of digoxin on mortality and morbidity in patients with heart failure. *N Engl J Med* 1997; 336:525-33.

Summary of drug management in chronic heart failure

Drug class	Potential therapeutic role
Diuretics	Symptomatic improvement of congestion. Spironolactone improves survival in severe (NYHA class IV) heart failure
Angiotensin converting enzyme (ACE) inhibitors	Improved symptoms, exercise capacity, and survival in patients with asymptomatic and symptomatic systolic dysfunction
Digoxin	Improved symptoms, exercise capacity, and fewer admissions to hospital
Angiotensin II receptor antagonists	Treatment of symptomatic heart failure in patients intolerant to ACE inhibitors*
Nitrates and hydralazine	Improved survival in symptomatic patients intolerant to ACE inhibitors or angiotensin II receptor antagonists*
β Blockers	Improved symptoms and survival in stable patients who are already receiving ACE inhibitors
Amiodarone	Prevention of arrhythmias in patients with symptomatic ventricular arrhythmias

*Recommendations of when these agents might be considered (the use of these agents has not been addressed in randomised trials of patients intolerant to ACE inhibitors).

The survival graph is adapted with permission from Doval et al (*Lancet* 1994;344:493-8). The table of inotropic drugs is adapted with permission from Niebauer et al (*Lancet* 1997;349:966). The table of results of a meta-analysis of effects of β blockers is adapted with permission from Lechat P et al (*Circulation* 1998;98:1184-91). The table on doses and titration of β blockers is adapted with permission from Remme WJ (*Eur Heart J* 1997;18:736-53).

9　Acute and chronic management strategies

T Millane, G Jackson, C R Gibbs, G Y H Lip

Acute and chronic management strategies in heart failure are aimed at improving both symptoms and prognosis, although management in individual patients will depend on the underlying aetiology and the severity of the condition. It is imperative that the diagnosis of heart failure is accompanied by an urgent attempt to establish its cause, as timely intervention may greatly improve the prognosis in selected cases—for example, in patients with severe aortic stenosis.

Management of acute heart failure

Assessment
Common presenting features include anxiety, tachycardia, and dyspnoea. Pallor and hypotension are present in more severe cases: the triad of hypotension (systolic blood pressure < 90 mm Hg), oliguria, and low cardiac output constitutes a diagnosis of cardiogenic shock. Severe acute heart failure and cardiogenic shock may be related to an extensive myocardial infarction, sustained cardiac arrhythmias (for example, atrial fibrillation or ventricular tachycardia), or mechanical problems (for example, acute papillary muscle rupture or postinfarction ventricular septal defect).

Severe acute heart failure is a medical emergency, and effective management requires an assessment of the underlying cause, improvement of the haemodynamic status, relief of pulmonary congestion, and improved tissue oxygenation. Clinical and radiographic assessment of these patients provides a guide to severity and prognosis: the Killip classification has been developed to grade the severity of acute and chronic heart failure.

Treatment
Basic measures should include sitting the patient in an upright position with high concentration oxygen delivered via a face mask. Close observation and frequent reassessment are required in the early hours of treatment, and patients with acute severe heart failure, or refractory symptoms, should be monitored in a high dependency unit. Urinary catheterisation facilitates accurate assessment of fluid balance, while arterial blood gases provide valuable information about oxygenation and acid-base balance. The "base excess" is a guide to actual tissue perfusion in patients with acute heart failure: a worsening (more negative) base excess generally indicates lactic acidosis, which is related to anaerobic metabolism, and is a poor prognostic feature. Correction of hypoperfusion will correct the metabolic acidosis; bicarbonate infusions should be reserved for only the most refractory cases.

Intravenous loop diuretics, such as frusemide (furosemide), induce transient venodilatation, when administered to patients with pulmonary oedema, and this may lead to symptomatic improvement even before the onset of diuresis. Loop diuretics also increase the renal production of vasodilator prostaglandins. This additional benefit is antagonised by the administration of prostaglandin inhibitors, such as non-steroidal anti-inflammatory drugs, and these agents should be avoided where possible. Parenteral opiates or opioids (morphine or diamorphine) are an important adjunct in the management of severe acute heart failure, by relieving anxiety, pain, and distress and reducing myocardial oxygen demand. Intravenous opiates

Survival rates (%) compared with chronic heart failure

	At 1 year	At 2 years	At 3 years
Breast cancer	88	80	72
Prostate cancer	75	64	55
Colon cancer	56	48	42
Heart failure	67	41	24

Killip classification

Class	Clinical features	Hospital mortality (%)
Class I	No signs of left ventricular dysfunction	6
Class II	S3 gallop with or without mild to moderate pulmonary congestion	30
Class III	Acute severe pulmonary oedema	40
Class IV	Shock syndrome	80-90

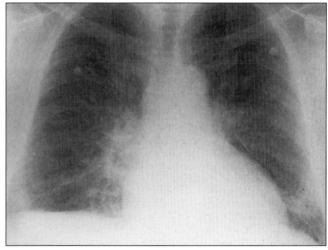
Chest *x* ray film in patient with acute pulmonary oedema

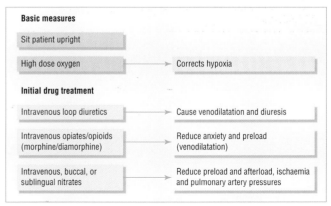
Acute heart failure: basic measures and initial drug treatment

and opioids also produce transient venodilatation, thus reducing preload, cardiac filling pressures, and pulmonary congestion.

Nitrates (sublingual, buccal, and intravenous) may also reduce preload and cardiac filling pressures and are particularly valuable in patients with both angina and heart failure. Sodium nitroprusside is a potent, directly acting vasodilator, which is normally reserved for refractory cases of acute heart failure.

Short term inotropic support

In cases of severe refractory heart failure in which the cardiac output remains critically low, the circulation can be supported for a critical period of time with inotropic agents. For example, dobutamine and dopamine have positive inotropic actions, acting on the β_1 receptors in cardiac muscle. Phosphodiesterase inhibitors (for example, enoximone) are less commonly used, and long term use of these agents is associated with increased mortality. Intravenous aminophylline is now rarely used for treating acute heart failure. Inotropic agents in general increase the potential for cardiac arrhythmias.

✈ Chronic heart failure

Chronic heart failure can be "compensated" or "decompensated." In compensated heart failure, symptoms are stable, and many overt features of fluid retention and pulmonary oedema are absent. Decompensated heart failure refers to a deterioration, which may present either as an acute episode of pulmonary oedema or as lethargy and malaise, a reduction in exercise tolerance, and increasing breathlessness on exertion. The cause or causes of decompensation should be considered and identified; they may include recurrent ischaemia, arrhythmias, infections, and electrolyte disturbance. Atrial fibrillation is common, and poor control of ventricular rate during exercise despite adequate control at rest should be addressed.

Common features of chronic heart failure include breathlessness and reduced exercise tolerance, and management is directed at relieving these symptoms and improving quality of life. Secondary but important objectives are to improve prognosis and reduce hospital admissions.

Initial management

Non-pharmacological and lifestyle measures should be addressed. Loop diuretics are valuable if there is evidence of fluid overload, although these may be reduced once salt and water retention has been treated. Angiotensin converting enzyme inhibitors should be introduced at an early stage, in the absence of clear contraindications. Angiotensin II receptor antagonists are an appropriate alternative in patients who are intolerant to angiotensin converting enzyme inhibitors. β Blockers (carvedilol, bisoprolol, metoprolol) are increasingly used in stable patients, although these agents require low dose initiation and cautious titration under specialist supervision. Oral digoxin has a role in patients with left ventricular systolic impairment, in sinus rhythm, who remain symptomatic despite optimal doses of diuretics and angiotensin converting enzyme inhibitors. Warfarin should be considered in patients with atrial fibrillation.

Severe congestive heart failure

Despite conventional treatment with diuretics and angiotensin converting enzyme inhibitors, hospital admission may be necessary in severe congestive heart failure. Fluid restriction is

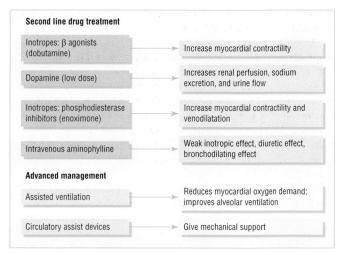

Acute heart failure: second line drug treatment and advanced management

---

Intravenous inotropes and circulatory assist devices
- Short term support with intravenous inotropes or circulatory assist devices, or with both, may temporarily improve haemodynamic status and peripheral perfusion
- Such support can act as a bridge to corrective valve surgery or cardiac transplantation in acute and chronic heart failure

---

Management of chronic heart failure

General advice
- Counselling—about symptoms and compliance
- Social activity and employment
- Vaccination (influenza, pneumococcal)
- Contraception

General measures
- Diet (for example, reduce salt and fluid intake)
- Stop smoking
- Reduce alcohol intake
- Take exercise

Treatment options—pharmacological
- Diuretics (loop and thiazide)
- Angiotensin converting enzyme inhibitors
- β Blockers
- Digoxin
- Spironolactone
- Vasodilators (hydralazine/nitrates)
- Anticoagulation
- Antiarrhythmic agents
- Positive inotropic agents

Treatment options—devices and surgery
- Revascularisation (percutaneous transluminal coronary angioplasty and coronary artery bypass graft)
- Valve replacement (or repair)
- Pacemaker or implantable cardiodefibrillator
- Ventricular assist devices
- Heart transplantation

Supervised exercise programmes are of proved benefit, and regular exercise should be encouraged in patients with chronic stable heart failure

important—fluid intake should be reduced to 1-1.5 litres/24 h, and dietary salt restriction may be helpful.

Short term bed rest is valuable until signs and symptoms improve: rest reduces the metabolic demand and increases renal perfusion, thus improving diuresis. Although bed rest potentiates the action of diuretics, it increases the risk of venous thromboembolism, and prophylactic subcutaneous heparin should be considered in immobile inpatients. Full anticoagulation is not advocated routinely unless concurrent atrial fibrillation is present, although it may be considered in patients with very severe impairment of left ventricular systolic function, associated with significant ventricular dilatation. Intravenous loop diuretics may be administered to overcome the short term problem of gut oedema and reduced absorption of tablets, and these may be used in conjunction with an oral thiazide or thiazide-like diuretic (metolazone). Low dose spironolactone (25 mg) improves morbidity and mortality in severe (New York Heart Association class IV) heart failure, when combined with conventional treatment (loop diuretics and angiotensin converting enzyme inhibitors). Potassium concentrations should be closely monitored after the addition of spironolactone.

Weighing the patient daily is valuable in monitoring the response to treatment

Education, counselling, and support
- A role is emerging for heart failure liaison nurses in educating and supporting patients and their families, promoting long term compliance, and supervising treatment changes in the community
- Depression is common, underdiagnosed, and often undertreated; counselling is therefore important for patients and families, and the newer antidepressants (particularly the selective serotonin reuptake inhibitors) seem to be well tolerated and are useful in selected patients

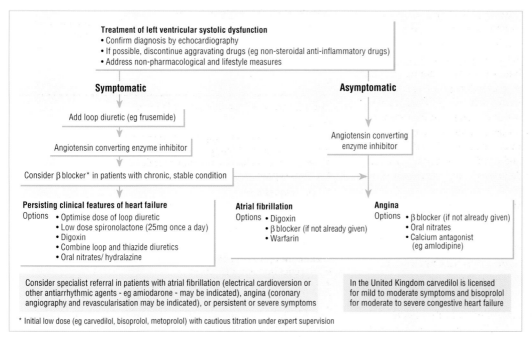

Treatment of left ventricular systolic dysfunction
- Confirm diagnosis by echocardiography
- If possible, discontinue aggravating drugs (eg non-steroidal anti-inflammatory drugs)
- Address non-pharmacological and lifestyle measures

Symptomatic / **Asymptomatic**

Add loop diuretic (eg frusemide)

Angiotensin converting enzyme inhibitor

Angiotensin converting enzyme inhibitor

Consider β blocker* in patients with chronic, stable condition

Persisting clinical features of heart failure
Options
- Optimise dose of loop diuretic
- Low dose spironolactone (25mg once a day)
- Digoxin
- Combine loop and thiazide diuretics
- Oral nitrates/ hydralazine

Atrial fibrillation
Options
- Digoxin
- β blocker (if not already given)
- Warfarin

Angina
Options
- β blocker (if not already given)
- Oral nitrates
- Calcium antagonist (eg amlodipine)

Consider specialist referral in patients with atrial fibrillation (electrical cardioversion or other antiarrhythmic agents - eg amiodarone - may be indicated), angina (coronary angiography and revascularisation may be indicated), or persistent or severe symptoms

In the United Kingdom carvedilol is licensed for mild to moderate symptoms and bisoprolol for moderate to severe congestive heart failure

* Initial low dose (eg carvedilol, bisoprolol, metoprolol) with cautious titration under expert supervision

Example of management algorithm for left ventricular dysfunction

Special procedures

Intra-aortic balloon pumping and mechanical devices
Intra-aortic balloon counterpulsation and left ventricular assist devices are used as bridges to corrective valve surgery, cardiac transplantation, or coronary artery bypass surgery in the presence of poor cardiac function. Mechanical devices are indicated if (a) there is a possibility of spontaneous recovery (for example, peripartum cardiomyopathy, myocarditis) or (b) as a bridge to cardiac surgery (for example, ruptured mitral papillary muscle, postinfarction ventricular septal defect) or transplantation. Intra-aortic balloon counterpulsation is the most commonly used form of mechanical support.

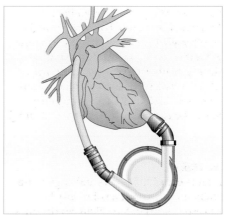

Left ventricular assist device

Revascularisation and other operative strategies

Impaired ventricular function in itself is not an absolute contraindication to cardiac surgery, although the operative risks are increased. Ischaemic heart disease is the most common precursor of chronic heart failure in Britain: coronary ischaemia should be identified and revascularisation considered with coronary artery bypass surgery or occasionally percutaneous coronary angioplasty. The concept of "hibernating" myocardium is increasingly recognised, although the most optimal and practical methods of identifying hibernation remain open to debate. Revascularisation of hibernating myocardium may lead to an improvement in the overall left ventricular function.

Correction of valve disease, most commonly in severe aortic stenosis or mitral incompetence (not secondary to left ventricular dilatation), relieves a mechanical cause of heart failure; closure of an acute ventricular septal defect or mitral valve surgery for acute mitral regurgitation, complicating a myocardial infarction, may be lifesaving. Surgical excision of a left ventricular aneurysm (aneurysectomy) is appropriate in selected cases. Novel surgical procedures such as extensive ventricular reduction (Batista operation) and cardiomyoplasty have been associated with successful outcome in a small number of patients, although the high mortality, and the limited evidence of substantial benefit, has restricted the widespread use of these procedures.

Cardiac transplantation

The outcome in cardiac transplantation is now good, with long term improvements in survival and quality of life in patients with severe heart failure. However, although the demand for cardiac transplantation has increased over recent years, the number of transplant operations has remained stable, owing primarily to limited availability of donor organs.

The procedure now carries a perioperative mortality of less than 10%, with approximate one, five, and 10 year survival rates of 92%, 75%, and 60% respectively (much better outcomes than with optimal drug treatment, which is associated with a one year mortality of 30-50% in advanced heart failure). Cardiac transplantation should be considered in patients with an estimated one year survival of <50%. Well selected patients over 55-60 years have a survival rate comparable to those of younger patients. Patients need strong social and psychological support; transplant liaison nurses are valuable in this role.

The long term survival of the transplanted human heart is compromised by accelerated graft atherosclerosis which results in small vessel coronary artery disease and an associated deterioration in left ventricular performance. This can occur as early as three months and is the major cause of graft loss after the first year. The anti-rejection regimens currently used may result in an acceleration of pre-existing atherosclerotic vascular disease—hence the exclusion of patients who already have significant peripheral vascular disease. Rejection is now a less serious problem, with the use of cyclosporin and other immunosuppressant agents.

Nevertheless, the supply of donors limits the procedure. The Eurotransplant database (1990-5) indicates that 25% of patients listed for transplantation die on the waiting list, with 60% receiving transplants at two years (most within 12 months). Although ventricular assist devices may be valuable during the wait for transplantation, the routine use of xenotransplants is unlikely in the short or medium term.

The graph showing cardiac transplantations worldwide is adapted with permission from Hosenpud et al (*J Heart Lung Transplant* 1998;17:656-8). The table showing survival rates is adapted from Hobbs (*Heart* 1999; 82(suppl IV):IV8-10).

Indications and contraindications to cardiac transplantation in adults

Indications
- End stage heart failure—for example, ischaemic heart disease and dilated cardiomyopathy
- Rarely, restrictive cardiomyopathy and peripartum cardiomyopathy
- Congenital heart disease (often combined heart-lung transplantation required)

Absolute contraindications
- Recent malignancy (other than basal cell and squamous cell carcinoma of the skin)
- Active infection (including HIV, Hepatitis B, Hepatitis C with liver disease)
- Systemic disease which is likely to affect life expectancy
- Significant pulmonary vascular resistance

Relative contraindications
- Recent pulmonary embolism
- Symptomatic peripheral vascular disease
- Obesity
- Severe renal impairment
- Psychosocial problems—for example, lack of social support, poor compliance, psychiatric illness
- Age (over 60-65 years)

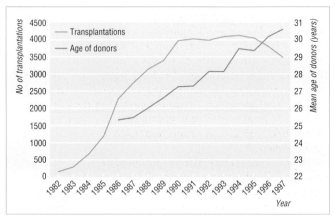

Number of heart transplantations worldwide and mean age of donors

Key references

- Dargie HJ, McMurray JJ. Diagnosis and management of heart failure. *BMJ* 1994;308:321-8.
- ACC/AHA Task Force Report. Guidelines for the evaluation and management of heart failure. *J Am Coll Cardiol* 1995;26:1376-98.
- Hunt SA. Current status of cardiac transplantation. *JAMA* 1998;280:1692-8.
- Remme WJ. The treatment of heart failure. The Task Force of the Working Group on Heart Failure of the European Society of Cardiology. *Eur Heart J* 1997;18:736-53.

10 Heart failure in general practice

F D R Hobbs, R C Davis, G Y H Lip

Management of heart failure in general practice has been hampered by difficulties in diagnosing the condition and by perceived difficulties in starting and monitoring treatment in the community. Nevertheless, improved access to diagnostic testing and increased confidence in the safety of treatment should help to improve the primary care management of heart failure. With improved survival and reduced admission rates (achieved by effective treatment) and a reduction in numbers of hospital beds, the community management of heart failure is likely to become increasingly important and the role of general practitioners even more crucial.

Diagnostic accuracy

Heart failure is a difficult condition to diagnose clinically, and hence many patients thought to have heart failure by their general practitioners may not have any demonstrable abnormality of cardiac function on objective testing.

A study from Finland reported that only 32% of patients suspected of having heart failure by primary care doctors had definite heart failure (as determined by a clinical and radiographic scoring system). A recent study in the United Kingdom showed that only 29% of 122 patients referred to a "rapid access" clinic with a new diagnosis of heart failure fully met the definition of heart failure approved by the European Society of Cardiology—that is, appropriate symptoms, objective evidence of cardiac dysfunction, and response to treatment if doubt remained.

Similar findings have been reported in the echocardiographic heart of England screening (ECHOES) study, in which only about 22% of the patients with a diagnosis of heart failure in their general practice records had definite impairment of left ventricular systolic function on echocardiography, with a further 16% having borderline impairment. In addition, 23% had atrial fibrillation, with over half of these patients having normal left ventricular systolic contraction. Finally, a minority of patients may have clinical heart failure with normal systolic contraction and abnormal diastolic function; management of such patients with diastolic dysfunction is very different from those with impaired systolic function.

Open access echocardiography and diagnosis

Owing to the non-invasive nature of echocardiography, its high acceptability to patients, and its usefulness in assessing ventricular size and function, as well as valvar heart disease, many general practitioners now want direct access to echocardiography services for their patients. Although open access echocardiography services are available in some districts in Britain, many specialists still have reservations about introducing such services because of financial and staffing issues and concern that general practitioners would have difficulty interpreting technical reports. The cost of echocardiography (£50 to £70 per patient) is relatively small, however, compared with the cost of expensive treatment for heart failure that may not be needed. The cost is also small compared with the costs of

Heart failure affects at least 20 patients on the average general practitioner's list

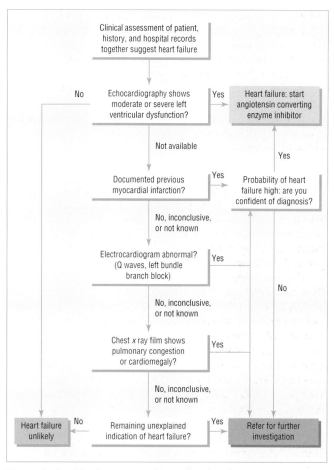

Diagnostic algorithm for suspected heart failure in primary care. Based on guidance from the north of England evidence based guideline development project (see key references box)

Recent studies have shown that with appropriate education of general practitioners the workload of an open access echocardiography service can be manageable

hospital admission, which may be avoided by appropriate, early treatment of heart failure.

One approach may be to refer only patients with abnormal baseline investigations as heart failure is unlikely if the electrocardiogram and chest x ray examination are normal and there are no predisposing factors for heart failure—for example, previous myocardial infarction, angina, hypertension, and diabetes mellitus. Requiring general practitioners to perform electrocardiography and arrange chest radiography, as a complement to careful assessment of the risk factors for heart failure, is likely to reduce substantially the number of inappropriate referrals to an open access echocardiography service.

Open access services have proved popular and are likely to become even more common; indeed, echocardiographic screening of patients in the high risk categories may well be justified and cost effective

Role of natriuretic peptides

Given the difficulties in diagnosing heart failure on clinical grounds alone, and current limited access to echocardiography and specialist assessment, the possibility of using a blood test in general practice to diagnose heart failure is appealing. Determining plasma concentrations of brain natriuretic peptide, a hormone found at an increased level in patients with left ventricular systolic dysfunction, may be one option. Such a blood test has the potential to screen out patients in whom heart failure is extremely unlikely and identify those in whom the probability of heart failure is high—for example, in patients with suspected heart failure who have low plasma concentrations of brain natriuretic peptide, the heart is unlikely to be the cause of the symptoms, whereas those who have higher concentrations warrant further assessment.

Sensitivity and specificity of brain natriuretic peptides in diagnosis of heart failure

	New diagnosis of heart failure (primary care)	Left ventricular systolic dysfunction
Sensitivity	97%	77%
Specificity	84%	87%
Positive predictive value	70%	16%

Primary prevention and early detection

General practitioners have a vital role in the early detection and treatment of the main risk factors for heart failure—namely, hypertension and ischaemic heart disease—and other cardiovascular risk factors, such as smoking and hyperlipidaemia. The Framingham study has shown a decline in hypertension as a risk factor for heart failure over the years, which probably reflects improvements in treatment. Ischaemic heart disease, however, remains very common. Aspirin, β blockers, and lipid lowering treatment, as well as smoking cessation, can reduce progression to myocardial infarction in patients with angina, and β blockers may also reduce ischaemic left ventricular dysfunction. Early detection of left ventricular dysfunction in "high risk" asymptomatic patients—for example, those who have already had a myocardial infarction or who have hypertension or atrial fibrillation—and treatment with angiotensin converting enzyme inhibitors can minimise the progression to symptomatic heart failure.

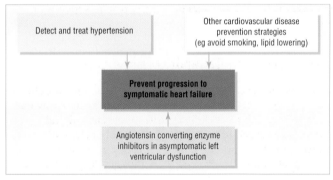

Strategies for preventing progression to symptomatic heart failure in high risk asymptomatic patients

Ⅹ Starting and monitoring drug treatment

Both hospital doctors and general practitioners used to be concerned about the initiation of angiotensin converting enzyme inhibitors outside hospital. It is now accepted, however, that most patients with heart failure can safely be established on such treatment without needing hospital admission. The previous concern—over first dose hypotension—was heightened by the initial experience of large doses of captopril, especially in those with severe heart failure, who are at greater risk of problems. Patients with mild or moderate heart failure, who have normal renal function and a systolic blood pressure over 100 mm Hg and who have stopped taking diuretics for at least 24 hours rarely have problems, especially if the first dose of an

Starting angiotensin converting enzyme inhibitors in chronic heart failure in general practice

- Measure blood pressure and determine electrolytes and creatinine concentrations before treatment
- Consider referring "high risk" patients to hospital for assessment and supervised start of treatment
- Angiotensin converting enzyme inhibitors should be used with some caution in patients with severe peripheral vascular disease because of the possible association with atherosclerotic renal artery stenosis
- Doses should be gradually increased over two to three weeks, aiming to reach the doses used in large clinical trials
- Blood pressure and electrolytes or renal chemistry should be monitored after start of treatment, initially at one week then less frequently depending on the patient and any abnormalities detected

angiotensin converting enzyme inhibitor is taken at night, before going to bed.

Heart failure clinics

Dedicated heart failure clinics within general practices, run by a doctor or nurse with an interest in the subject, have the potential to improve the care of patients with the condition, as they have for other chronic conditions, such as diabetes.

Blood should be taken for electrolytes and renal chemistry at least every 12 months, but more frequently in new cases and when drug treatment has been changed or results have been abnormal. The clinics should be used to educate patients about their condition, particularly in relation to their treatment, with messages being reinforced and drug treatment simplified and rationalised where appropriate. Patients whose condition is deteriorating may be referred for specialist opinion.

Variables that should be monitored in patients with established heart failure comprise changes in symptoms and severity (New York Heart Association classification); weight; blood pressure; and signs of fluid retention or excessive diuresis.

Impact of heart failure on the community

After a patient is diagnosed as having heart failure, substantial monitoring by the general practitioner is required. In our survey of heart failure in three general practices from the west of Birmingham, 44% of general practice consultations (average 2.6 visits per patient) took place within three months of the first diagnosis of heart failure, 23% were at three to six months (1.4 visits per patient), and 33% were at six to 12 months (2.0 visits per patient). Such management requires regular supervision and audit.

Relevance to hospital practice

In our survey of acute hospital admissions of patients with heart failure to a city centre hospital, the median duration of stay was 8 (range 1-96) days, with 20% inpatient mortality. Clinical variables associated with an adverse prognosis include the presence of atrial fibrillation, poor exercise tolerance, electrolyte abnormalities, and the presence of coronary artery disease. Angiotensin converting enzyme inhibitors were prescribed in only 51% of heart failure patients on discharge; after the first diagnosis of heart failure, the average number of hospital attendances (inpatient and outpatient) in the first 12 months was 3.2 visits per patient, with an average of 6.0 general practice consultations per patient. However, 44% of hospital attendances (1.4 visits per patient) took place within three months of diagnosis, 33% were at three to six months (1.0 visits per patient), and 23% were at 6-12 months (0.74 visits per patient).

These figures represent the collective burden of heart failure on hospital practice. Indeed, about 200 000 people in the United Kingdom require admission to hospital for heart failure each year.

Specialist nurse support

The important role of nurses in the management of heart failure has been relatively neglected in Britain. In the United States the establishment of a nurse managed heart failure clinic in South Carolina resulted in a reduction in readmissions of 4%

Conditions indicating that referral to a specialist is necessary

- Diagnosis in doubt or when specialist investigation and management may help
- Significant murmurs and valvar heart disease
- Arrhythmias—for example, atrial fibrillation
- Secondary causes—for example, thyroid disease
- Severe left ventricular impairment—for example, ejection fraction <20%
- Pre-existing (or developing) metabolic abnormalities—for example, hyponatraemia (sodium <130 mmol/l) and renal impairment
- Severe associated vascular disease—for example, caution with angiotensin converting enzyme inhibitors in case of coexisting renovascular disease
- Relative hypotension (systolic blood pressure <100 mm Hg before starting angiotensin converting enzyme inhibitors)
- Poor response to treatment

Examples of topics for audit of heart failure management in general practice

Means of diagnosis
Has left ventricular function been assessed, by echocardiography or other means?

Appropriateness of treatment
Are all appropriate patients taking angiotensin converting enzyme inhibitors (unless there is a documented contraindication)? Have doses been increased where possible to those used in the large clinical trials?

Monitoring treatment
Were blood pressure and renal function recorded before and after start of angiotensin converting enzyme inhibitors, and at intervals subsequently?

Causes of readmission in patients with heart failure

- Angina
- Infections
- Arrhythmias
- Poor compliance
- Inadequate drug treatment
- Iatrogenic factors
- Inadequate discharge planning or follow up
- Poor social support

Admissions with heart failure over six months to a district general hospital serving a multiracial population

Presentation (%)	Associated medical history (%)
Pulmonary oedema (52)	Ischaemic heart disease (54)
Congestive heart failure, with fluid overload (32)	Hypertension (34)
Myocardial infarction and heart failure (9)	Valve disease (12); previous stroke (10)
Associated atrial fibrillation (29)	Diabetes mellitus (19); peripheral vascular disease (13); cardiomyopathy (1)

Population of 300 000 (7451 admissions; 348 (5%) had heart failure (mean age 73 years)).

and in length of hospital stay of almost two days. In another North American study a comprehensive, multidisciplinary approach to heart failure management, including supervision by nurses, resulted in a significant (56%) reduction in readmissions and hospital stay, with a trend towards reduced mortality. Quality of life scores also improved in the intervention group. A more dramatic result was obtained in a study from Adelaide, Australia, where multidisciplinary intervention resulted in a 20% reduction in mortality.

Nurse management of heart failure has implications for the provision of care in patients with chronic heart failure, sharing the increasing burden of heart failure. Specialist nurses would provide advice, information, and support to patients with heart failure and to their families and would ensure that the best treatment is given. The potential benefits are substantial, with reduced hospital admission rates, improved quality of life, and lower costs.

Economic considerations

With an increasingly elderly population, the prevalence of heart failure could have increased by as much as 70% by the year 2010. Heart failure currently accounts for 1-2% of total spending on health care in Europe and in the United States. In 1993 in the United Kingdom, heart failure cost the NHS £360m a year; the figure now is probably closer to £600m, equivalent to 1-2% of the total NHS budget, and hospital admissions account for 60-70% of this expenditure. Admissions for heart failure have been increasing and are expected to increase further. Preventing disease progression, hence reducing the frequency and duration of admissions, is therefore an important objective in the treatment of heart failure in the future.

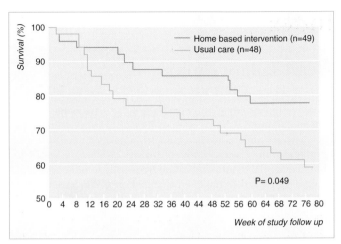

Cumulative survival curves from the Adelaide nurse intervention study: 18 month follow up (see Stewart et al, key references box at end of article)

Economic cost of heart failure to NHS in UK, 1990-1

	Total cost (£m)	% of total cost
General practice visits	8.3	2.5
Referrals to hospital from general practice	8.2	2.4
Other outpatient attendances	31.8	9.4
Inpatient stay	213.8	63.5
Diagnostic tests	45.6	13.5
Drugs	22.1	6.6
Surgery	7.2	2.1
Total	337.0	100

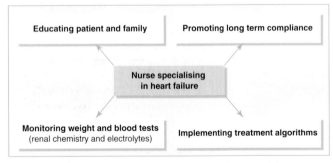

Role of specialist nurse in management of patients with heart failure

Heart failure is likely to continue to become a major public health problem in the coming decades; new and better management strategies are necessary, including risk factor interventions, for patients at risk of developing heart failure

The table on sensitivity and specificity is based on information in Cowie et al (*Lancet* 1997;350:1349-53) and McDonagh et al (*Lancet* 1998;351:9-13). The table showing admissions with heart failure to a district general hospital is adapted with permission from Lip et al (*Int J Clin Prac* 1997;51: 223-7). The table showing the economic costs of heart failure is published with permission from McMurray et al (*Eur Heart J* 1993;14(suppl):133).

Key references

- Eccles M, Freemantle N, Mason J, for the North of England Guideline Development Group. North of England evidence based development project: guideline for angiotensin converting enzyme inhibitors in primary care management of adults with symptomatic heart failure. *BMJ* 1998;316:1369-75.
- Francis CM, Caruana L, Kearney P, Love M, Sutherland GR, Starkey IR, et al. Open access echocardiography in the management of heart failure in the community. *BMJ* 1995;310:634-6.
- Lip GYH, Sarwar S, Ahmed I, Lee S, Kapoor V, Child D, et al. A survey of heart failure in general practice. The west Birmingham heart failure project. *Eur J Gen Pract* 1997;3:85-9.
- Remes J, Miettinen H, Reunanen A, Pyorala K. Validity of clinical diagnosis of heart failure in primary health care. *Eur Heart J* 1991;12:315-21.
- Rich MW, Beckham V, Wittenberg C, Leven CL, Freedland KE, Carney RM, et al. A multidisciplinary intervention to prevent the readmission of elderly patients with congestive heart failure. *N Engl J Med* 1995:333:1190-5.
- Stewart S, Vandenbroek AJ, Pearson S, Horowitz JD. Prolonged beneficial effects of home-based intervention on unplanned readmissions and mortality among patients with congestive heart failure. *Arch Intern Med* 1999;159:257-61.

Index